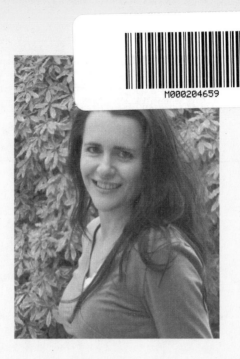

Melinda Tankard Reist is an Australian writer and researcher with a special interest in bioethics, women's health and medical abuses of women. She trained and worked as a journalist in Victoria and was awarded a Rotary Foundation Scholarship to study journalism in the United States. Melinda's work has been published in newspapers and journals, and broadcast on radio programs, in Australia and overseas. Melinda has worked as a political adviser; she is a founding director of Women's Forum Australia, an independent women's think tank, and is also involved in advocacy and support for pregnant women.

Also by Melinda Tankard Reist

Giving Sorrow Words: Women's Stories of Grief After Abortion
    (2000)

DEFIANT BIRTH

WOMEN WHO RESIST MEDICAL EUGENICS

Melinda Tankard Reist

Spinifex Press Pty Ltd
504 Queensberry Street
North Melbourne, Vic. 3051
Australia
women@spinifexpress.com.au
http://www.spinifexpress.com.au

First published 2006
Copyright © Melinda Tankard Reist
Copyright on all contributions belongs to authors unless otherwise indicated
Copyright on layout, Spinifex Press, 2006
Any copyright holders not acknowledged here or acknowledged incorrectly
should contact the publishers.

Edited and indexed by Kerry Biram
Cover design by Deb Snibson
Typeset by Claire Warren
Printed and bound by McPherson's Printing Group

National Library of Australia cataloguing-in-publication data:

Tankard Reist, Melinda.
Defiant birth : women who resist medical eugenics.

  Bibliography.
  Includes index.
  ISBN 1 876756 59 4.

  1. Eugenics. 2. Pregnancy – Complications. 3. Women
  with Disabilities. 4. Fetus – Abnormalities. I. Title.

363.920994

To the women whose experiences became this book.

Contents

Acknowledgements

First, to Philippa, who lit the spark for this book and contributed significant preliminary work (including the website http://defiantbirth.com) to start it on its way, thank you so much. Deepest gratitude to Renate Klein and Susan Hawthorne for saying "Yes!" when the proposal wasn't much more than a two-word title, *Defiant Birth*. Your guidance, support and encouragement have meant so much. Thanks for believing in this book. Ros and Kate – significant appreciation (it's over now!). To John, heartfelt thanks for suggestions (and for once more lending me your home in which to write); Michael, for your obsessive-compulsive attention to detail and gracious support; Selena and Greg for generous assistance, especially with locating obscure reference material and for help with the glossary; Warwick, Christopher, Jeremy, Lynne and Katrina for helpful comments. To Belinda Morris at Spinifex for calm checking and unflagging enthusiasm for the book and Kerry Biram for editing. And to all the contributors for your generosity in sharing your stories here. To David, Ariel, Jordan, Kelsey and Layla for seeing me through another book.

. . . he detected where destiny beckoned. The future for babies like him never looked more promising, but now society frowned upon giving spastic babies a right to life. Now they threatened to abort babies like him, to detect in advance their handicapped state, to burrow through the womb and label them for death, to baffle their mothers with fear for their coming . . .

From Christopher Nolan's autobiography,
Under the Eye of the Clock (1987, p. 119).

Is the story claiming that the pregnancy has malfunctioned . . . resulting in a baby with a malformation, any 'truer' than the story suggesting that society has malfunctioned because it cannot accommodate the disabled in its midst?

From Abby Lippman, Prenatal genetic testing and screening:
Constructing needs and reinforcing inequities (1991, p. 44).

Introduction

Defiant Birth is a book about women who have resisted the present day practice of medical eugenics. It is about women who were told they should not have babies because of perceived disabilities – either in the child or themselves. They have confronted a society deeply fearful of disability and all its stigmas.[1] Facing silent disapproval and even open hostility, they have had their babies anyway, believing their children are just as worthy to partake of life as are others.

This is a book about women who have resisted the ideology of quality control and the paradigm of perfection. They have dared to challenge the prevailing medical and social mindset. This book's contributors have refused to take part in a system of disability deselection (Wolbring, 2003) which classifies certain people as biologically incapacitated (Spallone, 1992, p. 180). These women may be among the last who decide to have babies without the genetic stamp of approval. They are, in a sense, genetic outlaws.[2]

Defiant Birth confronts the widespread medical, and often-times social, aversion to less-than-perfect pregnancies or genetically different babies. Some women who contacted me were confronted with extraordinary objections to their desire to proceed with their pregnancies. One American woman, pregnant at 46 with triplets, was rejected for care by twelve doctors. Others were abandoned by medical practitioners when they declined 'the standard of care' on offer: termination. Still more were disparaged and treated as pariahs for departing from accepted medical wisdom about becoming pregnant at all.

A disturbing number of women in this book (and others whose stories don't appear here) were given grave diagnoses for their babies – regaled with a litany of abnormalities and 'life-threatening' conditions. But their babies were born without the predicted problems or with lesser difficulties. This raises questions about the accuracy of screening procedures and the clearly ill-placed faith in their veracity. How many women are being forced to make agonising decisions on the basis of inadequate – even inaccurate – information?

The medical establishment seems to be asking women to ratify social prejudice by subjecting them to a raft of screening technologies. The main purpose of these technologies is to weed out those babies deemed unsuitable, 'bad babies'[3] and not the 'blue ribbon babies'[4] they were meant to be. The profession urges women to quest for a 'better endowed' (Rakowski, 2002) child than the one they now carry; to eliminate 'worthless life' and replace it with a 'worthwhile life' (Glover, 1990).

Screening has become so routine and entrenched that many women are not aware that essentially the only 'therapy' to treat any problems found – or thought to be found – in the baby, is abortion.[5] Screening and abortion are routine procedures for 'baby-making' today.[6]

While more genetic screening now takes place during pregnancy and the newborn period than at any other time, many women report they don't even know why they are having the tests. A review based on 106 publications from 12 countries (Green et al., 2004) found that women's understanding of screening was poor and that most women were not making informed choices about undergoing screening.

In reading and considering the stories of the women in this

book, we need to look at the larger landscape which makes 'defiant birth' stand out. This Introduction therefore examines their stories in the broader framework of the use of technology including prenatal genetic diagnosis (PGD), the attitudes of the medical profession towards screening and abortion, limits to the notion of 'choice', eugenic thinking from the pre-war era and its influence on medical practice today, the rise of genetic consumerism, what it means to be a woman with a disability who wants to be a mother, and the language, euphemisms and strategies employed to get women and babies to conform to a specific medical and social model of perfection.

In the Afterword, I will consider the struggle of those with a disability to find adequate resources and care, the erosion of empathy and how these technologies and the quest for perfection could be changing the whole meaning of what it is to be human.

The medical gaze

Eugenically influenced medical advice appears to have become the norm, though it may not be recognised as such. The practices outlined in this book are part of what has been described as 'the infiltration and immense power of medicalization during routine pregnancy care' (Markens et al., 1999, p. 368).

Even healthy women are made to feel there could be something very wrong medically with their pregnancy. A friend, healthy and pregnant with child number three, told me she was encouraged to have a nuchal translucency screen to test for Down syndrome because, 'after all, you are 27'. Fewer and fewer pregnancies are allowed to proceed without screening and related interventions. Rarely are women allowed to move through pregnancy without being subjected to some form of genetic surveillance. Some of the drive to 'over-screen' is driven by medical negligence claims; doctors, and no less their insurers, push for routine screening as a means of ensuring that their risk of liability is minimised.[7] Finlay et al., quoting Margrit Shildrick, observe:

> In prenatal care, the reductive view of the body associated with this necessary focus on competency has led to a 'medical gaze' in which women are discursively constructed as 'baby machines' (Shildrick, 1997, p. 22) whose products are faulty, rather than women who are very connected both emotionally and physically to the process of pregnancy (Finlay et al., 2004, p. 15).

This medical gaze becomes even sharper when focussing on women who may be 'at risk' of avoiding screening. Women are often led to infer that it is only those who are weak-willed and avoidance-seeking who do not avail themselves of all medical technology has to offer. As Alice Wexler points out:

> Clinician led counselling for PGT [prenatal genetic testing] in such a discursive framework is permeated with the notion that to be tested is 'courageous' while not being tested is 'denial' and a wish to 'avoid' the truth. The clinical discourse also mobilises the concept of risk as a strategy for normalising the increasing use of the technology for most pregnancies and the concept of widened reproductive choice to authorize its incursions into healthy pregnancies (in Finlay et al., 2004, p. 15).[8]

'I was thought of as totally selfish for not finding out if my baby was perfect or not,' writes Diana Aldrich in the second story in this book.

Genetic screening in context: Towards a eugenics civilization

The practice of prenatal screening cannot be seen in isolation. It should be considered in the context of rapidly advancing reproductive technologies and genetic engineering developments such as in-vitro fertilisation, surrogacy, sperm donation (sought especially from those with high IQs) and the sale of 'eugenically superior' eggs,[9] embryo freezing, pre-implantation genetic diagnosis, genetic testing and sex-selection of embryos and experiments on aborted foetuses and foetal tissue transplants.[10]

Add to this the Human Genome Project, DNA chips, human reproductive and so-called 'therapeutic' cloning, the harvesting of stem cells from human embryos, gene therapy and now 'biobanks'. Genetic engineering of human eggs and sperm and 'germinal choice technology' involving genetic interventions to customise and 'improve' our children, are not all that far over the horizon.

As the prominent writer on science, technology and culture, Jeremy Rifkin says, these technologies are 'paving the way for the wholesale alteration of the human species and the birth of a commercially driven eugenics civilization . . .' (Rifkin, 1998, pp. 9, 28; see also Hawthorne, 2002).

Diversity is upheld as a value, yet great efforts are made to ensure that certain mothers don't have children, and that certain children are never to be allowed to contribute to this diversity. In this sense, at least, humanity is becoming increasingly homogenous. Babies born outside a standard view of what is normative are viewed as muddying the gene pool and costing the 'normal' citizens of society too much money. The stories in this book should raise concerns in our minds about 'biological pluralism and the elimination of genetic variations'.[11]

Kathy Evans, who won an award for 'Tuesday's child', a magazine article about her third child who was born with Down syndrome, reflects:

> Perhaps mine are the misshapen memories of youth, but as a child I saw more people with Down syndrome than I do today. I worry that by the time Caoimhe emerges into adulthood children like her will be gone forever (Evans, 2003, p. 4).[12]

Some doctors are already working to ensure this is exactly what will happen. Australian obstetrician Dr Andrew McLennan is very happy with nuchal translucency screening because 'Now we've got a system that allows us to pick up close to 85 per cent or 90 per cent [of babies with Down syndrome]. So that's a significant improvement in a short space of time' (Swan, 2001).

Genetic screeners and engineers hold significant power over human life, determining which human body gets the stamp of approval and which does not. As Christopher Nolan is quoted as saying at the beginning of this book, they decide who is 'labelled for death'. It seems we are reaching a point (or going back to a time?) when only those of suitable genetic merit and physical constitution are deemed worthy to have passed the test that allows them to participate in life.

Where once the disabled were shunted off to institutions to be hidden away, now screening with termination plays the same role. Says Barbara Field in a 1996 lecture: 'surely termination is the ultimate in concealment' (in Fitzgerald, 2005).

Prenatal diagnosis has become accepted as almost a ritual in pregnancy and is now 'the most widespread application of genetic technology to humans today' (Lippman, 1991, p. 19).

US philosopher Leon Kass, whose article 'The moral meaning of genetic technology' should be read by anyone concerned about where we are heading, observes that

> [N]ot only are they [scientists, doctors] creating life, but they stand in judgement of each being's worthiness to live or die (genetic screening and abortion) – not on moral grounds . . . but on somatic and genetic ones; they also hold out the promise of salvation from our genetic sins and defects (gene therapy and genetic engineering) (Kass, 1999, p. 35).

Kass relates an experience at his own university – Chicago – in which

> [A] physician making rounds with medical students stood over the bed of an intelligent, otherwise normal ten-year-old boy with spina bifida. 'Were he to have been conceived today,' the physician casually informed his entourage, 'he would have been aborted.' Determining who shall live and who shall die – on the basis of genetic merit – is a godlike power already wielded by genetic medicine. This power will only grow (Kass, 1999, p. 35).[13]

It is important to point out that many more children become disabled at or shortly after birth than those who had a disability before they were born. Moreover, people who acquire disabilities in later life such as in adolescence and adulthood vastly outnumber those who develop a condition as children. As Lisa Blumberg (1994b) has observed, disability is an inherent part of the human condition.

Lack of choice and the coercive power of testing

What does so-called 'freedom of choice' mean in a society where choices have become so prescribed, where there are fewer and fewer opportunities to opt out, where it is becoming harder to say 'No' to certain technologies and the expectations which automatically flow from their application? What does 'choice' mean when mothers are made to feel 'baffled with fear for [their babies'] coming' (Nolan, 1987, p. 119), where those who do go against what is expected of them and have, for example, a child with Down syndrome, are asked, 'But didn't you have the test?'

As Tom Shakespeare, who has a disability, argues: '. . . in hundreds of small ways, the choice is unfree, and the dice are loaded against the birth of disabled children' (Shakespeare, 1999, p. 30). Rather than opening up choices, prenatal screening could ultimately be shutting them down. Barbara Katz Rothman puts it succinctly:

> The introduction of that choice [to screen] may ultimately cost us the choice not to control the quality, the choice of taking our chances in life's great, glorious, and terrifying roll of the hundred thousand dice (Rothman, 1998, p. 287).

This view is echoed by Jane Hall, Rosalie Viney, and Marion Haas, who point out: 'Once an intervention is available, it tends to be used so that the range of what is accepted as normal is decreased' (Hall et al., 1998, p. 757). Anne Finger (1990, p. 42) concurs: '. . . social pressure can work to keep people in line . . . when a technology is available it becomes harder and harder not to utilize it.'

Over a third of obstetricians surveyed in England and Wales say that they generally require a woman to agree to terminate an affected pregnancy before they do prenatal diagnosis. A total of 13 per cent agreed with the statement: 'The state should not be expected to pay for the specialised care of a child with a severe handicap where the parents had declined the offer of prenatal diagnosis of the handicap' (Green, 1995, p. 102).

Indeed, many women do not experience prenatal diagnoses as a choice, but as a standard medical directive. Their autonomy is undermined when society determines which choices they are to be offered and makes them feel irresponsible for not exercising one of these pre-determined 'right' choices. Pressure placed on women who refuse to co-operate with the screening system is 'a dangerous assault on women's bodily autonomy' (Finger, 1990, p. 42).

Testing creates its own imperative to act on the results. One woman has said, 'If they'd handed her to me and said she was Down's I'd have been upset but I'd have got on with it; but once you've got into the testing trap you have to get to the end' (in

Statham and Green, 1993, p. 175).

The pressure to undergo screening has dire repercussions for those whose child is born with some type of impairment. Because of the widespread availability of testing – and due to burgeoning health care costs – those parents who have such a child are considered irresponsible either if they failed to avail themselves of the tests or if they ignored the findings. And because it was their decision to have such a child, the reasoning goes that they shouldn't expect everyone else to help them care for that child.[14]

In *The future of the disabled in liberal society*, Hans S. Reinders points to where this attitude could take us:

> Once the assumption of individual responsibility for the reproduction of 'bad genes' is firmly in place, people will be wary of sharing the costs of health care services for people with special needs whose existence they believe to be caused by 'irresponsible reproductive behaviour' (Reinders, 2000, pp. 85–86, 90).

If the treatment of women who have had one child with a disability when they could have availed themselves of the selection/abortion package is of concern, then consider the plight of women who have had more than one child with the same condition. Sam Tormey, writing in the *Griffith Review* (Australia) relates the experience of a woman he calls Sarah D. who was berated by a 'shocked' and 'open mouthed' bystander who said: 'Not one . . . not one but two. Don't you know that kind of thing is preventable now?' (Tormey, 2004).

The routinisation of testing

When something is accepted as *just routine*, fewer questions are asked about it. Informed decision making falls by the wayside (Green and Statham, 1996, p. 143).

In their examination of a Californian screening program, Nancy

Press and C. H. Browner exposed what they call a pro-testing 'institutional culture' within the program. They found screening was embedded into routine prenatal care, delivered as a 'standard package' (Press and Browner, 1997). Frequent meetings took place to check staff compliance with the state Maternal Serum Alpha Fetoprotein [AFP] mandate. Memos highlighted the need to develop an 'AFP consciousness' (Press and Browner, 1993). '. . . [R]outinisation of innovations often follows a trajectory that confounds or appears to obviate the need for systematic evaluation' they write (Press and Browner, 1997, p. 979).

Even the established principle of informed consent was considered negotiable:

> So strong was the presumption in these studies that testing was both good and unproblematic that all issues of informed consent – including whether informed consent was even necessary – were left to the discretion of the investigators at each research site (Press and Browner, 1997, p. 981).

The studies revealed how the issues of eugenics, disability and abortion were obscured in this 'routinisation'. This in turn helped achieve a high level of test acceptance. There was a 'purposeful ignoring' of the connection between prenatal testing and abortion. Nurses rarely mentioned abortion when discussing screening with a couple and the official state booklet on AFP given to all eligible women didn't even mention the word. Susan Markens et al. comment:

> Downplaying the relationship between fetal screening and abortion encouraged women to accept the test because it allowed them to think about it simply as an ordinary part of prenatal medical care.[15] The vast majority of women were negative or deeply conflicted about the idea of terminating their baby for fetal anomalies, particularly in the second trimester (1999, p. 362).

As the same authors observe:

> . . . agreeing to this screening did not truly constitute a decision
> . . . it was presented as the medically and maternally responsible
> course of action (Markens et al., 1999, p. 362).

As one woman commented on her own experience of screening, 'I have the principle that all the tests which are done are done for my and my baby's best interests. It was self-evident to participate' (in Santalahti et al., 1998, p. 1070).

Presenting the AFP screening test as merely a simple blood test, 'pulls all pregnant women into the world of prenatal testing and, concomitantly, into the world of "risk" associated with it' (Markens et al., 1999, p. 366).

The shock women are in for when they are not fully informed of a connection between screening and abortion can be devastating. One couple were not properly apprised of what being scheduled for an 'induction' really meant. They didn't realise what it involved until they got to the labour ward. In their own words:

> It was like we were in a tunnel and there was only one way out. I just didn't think that I had any choice but to go with what was suggested. I don't understand why they didn't discuss all the options. I don't think that we thought of the consequences of what we were doing. I went in to have the baby induced – that was the word used. It didn't register with us that they were going to terminate the pregnancy (in Beech & Anderson, 1999, p. 253).[16]

A number of women have told me that medical professionals tried to assure them the procedure was not really an abortion, but merely 'bringing on the birth'.

Natalie Withers was also not prepared for what she would go through with the late termination of her fourth daughter, whom she named Dellaney. The baby was diagnosed in 2001 with heart problems and a condition causing her stomach and liver to reverse.

When I spoke with Natalie (13 May 2005), she told me the procedure only had been discussed with her on the day she was due to be induced. She was told there would be two pills put into her cervix to induce labour and that it could take a few hours. Natalie says she ended up being administered eight to ten pills. Labour began on a Monday, and the baby was not delivered until Wednesday.

It was only when she was in labour that it was explained to her that the baby might either be stillborn or might take a breath immediately after the birth. Natalie recalls:

> I didn't realise at 20 weeks I would be handed a little person . . . The nurse said, 'Do you want to look because it's not that nice [due to the damage done to the body during the induced labour]?' They put clothes on her but didn't wipe the blood off first, the clothes were stuck to the blood. A quick glimpse, and they took her away. Had we been encouraged to, we would have held her. We said no to an autopsy because we didn't want them to touch her. Against our wishes, they did an autopsy and I had to go in to the hospital for the post-mortem report.

In retrospect Natalie realises she had 'massive reservations' about an abortion and feels she wasn't given time or space to air them. 'A big part of the weight I carried was that we had to sign her life away. I would still have grieved at her dying [if we didn't abort and she died after birth], but I wouldn't be carrying the same weight. The burden you carry is too great.'

Natalie has since learnt more about her daughter's condition and discovered that children with this condition can survive and do well with the right care. She carries with her a newspaper article about a child with the same condition who is now three.[17]

The right to choose not to know

It appears that the right-not-to-know the health status of one's foetus through prenatal testing is being daily eroded. To not want to be tested, or to not want to know what may turn up during an ultrasound screen, is to be considered irrational. One woman told me she specifically stated before her ultrasound that she did not want to know of any negative findings. On taking the ultrasound photo home to show her family she discovered to her shock a number of possible abnormalities written down the side. (The baby was later born free of any of these conditions.)

Henriikka Clarkeburn believes that '[a] duty to acquire information about the genetic constitution of the fetus must be connected to a duty to act upon that information' (2000, p. 400).[18] Kapuscinski and Popper also believe there is a duty to know. '. . . [I]gnorance has an ethical dimension, and knowing is a moral obligation for human beings' (Kapuscinski & Popper, 1995, p. 24).[19]

Kelly Jensen would be condemned by these commentators. She rejected the AFP test because of the negative repercussions that might result. As she put it: 'I have my reasons for not having certain testing . . . An unnecessary anxiety in a lot of cases. I think that it can [cause anxiety] rather than reassure' (in Markens et al., 1999, p. 364). Similarly, Lucille, an Australian-born rural woman expecting her first child, said of her refusal of prenatal tests: 'We felt that the information, if negative, if we did have the test, would cause unnecessary anxiety through the pregnancy' (in Liamputtong et al., 2003, p. 99).

'Brenda' reflects this feeling of being made to feel irresponsible when she comments: 'That's the bad part: that people can say to you, "You didn't have the tests?" or "Why didn't you have the tests?" You have to justify why you've brought a disabled child into the world!' (in Brookes, 1998, p. 304).

Libby Strahan would also be criticised for 'choosing ignorance'.

Because screening ruined her experience of pregnancy the first time around, the next time she chose not to know. In a letter to the editor in *The Age* newspaper in Melbourne, Australia, she wrote:

> I question the idea that early diagnosis for *all* pregnant women is helpful. It is only of real value if the parents will terminate; foetal treatments are rare.
>
> After two healthy daughters our unborn son was diagnosed abnormal at a routine ultrasound. We were told information would help us 'prepare'. This was our preparation: months of grief!
>
> We tried to lower our girls' expectations of a healthy baby. We changed to a bigger hospital and had more ultrasounds and consultations. Some ultrasounds were made difficult by my shaking – from sobbing. I bought no clothes for him, as these don't fit around tubes.
>
> After all this angst he was stillborn and we were relieved. Just because we didn't want a disabled child didn't mean we could terminate him. The only time our son lived was inside me, and we lost all joy in that for the last four months. If we were to have a disabled child we have the rest of our lives to get used to it – why start before you can even hold them?
>
> The next pregnancy, as two educated professionals, we chose ignorance and were delighted with both the pregnancy and another healthy daughter (Strahan, 2003, p. 12).

Finlay et al. describe the way in which '. . . logic has become regarded as a good in itself, producing a discourse around PGT [prenatal genetic testing] in which all information is considered to be desirable, those who opt not to know the genetic status of their unborn child are considered irrational' (2004, p. 15). Michael Taussig (1992) sets these attitudes within a context he describes as 'the fetishism of medicine'.

For many women, being pulled into the world of prenatal testing leads to their own desires being ignored; they are not considered relevant. A case study in *Nursing Ethics*, titled 'We went through psychological hell', provides evidence of the way women's own wishes are circumvented. It tells, for example, the experience of Barbara, a bioethics student, aware of the risks of amniocentesis, who wished to proceed with her pregnancy. But this wasn't taken into account. '. . . none of this counted as history worth documenting' (in Beech and Anderson, 1999, p. 250).[20]

Gwen Anderson writes about the repercussions when medical professionals do not take into account a couple's values and beliefs:

> When spouses are not given the opportunity to articulate differences, similarities or puzzling paradoxes that arise, their values, beliefs and moral convictions may remain less than fully explored . . . What is most important, what is at stake, what distinguishes rational thinking from overwhelming emotions, and what constitutes ethical quandaries or moral uncertainty is all too often left unspoken or misunderstood (Anderson, 1999, p. 131).

Language used to describe an individual's moral views is often 'brushed aside or invalidated on the grounds that it is non reasoned thinking, or it is emotion based, or it is unchallenged religious dogma' (Anderson, 1999, p. 134).

Alison Streeter's experience with a counsellor in a Sydney genetics clinic, as told in this book, is another example of how objections to the counsellor's recommended course of action are undermined as emotional and/or 'religious', that is, not rational and sensible.

Thomas Faunce, of the Australian National University, writing in the *Journal of Law and Medicine*, discusses the example of a woman who refuses a screening test. The woman says that under the common law in New South Wales (Australia) it is illegal for the doctor to offer abortion for any foetal condition which is not a danger to her physical or mental health. She says that this 'attempted coercion . . . into genetic screening' is 'a eugenic invasion of her privacy' and 'questions the idiosyncratic and unchallenged manner in which doctors can dress up such a political determination as a purely medical decision' (in Faunce, 1998, p. 148).

Eugenic invasions of privacy are common experiences of the women in this book. They too encounter doctors dressing up political determinations based on their own notions of perfectionism as purely medical decisions.

The 'benevolent tyranny of expertise'

As the stories in this book show, women are expected to place all their trust in the medical profession and in screening tests. It is not easy to stand up to the view of 'doctor knows best'. Leon Kass makes a pertinent point about the power carried by doctors:

> While a small portion of the population may be sufficiently educated to participate knowingly and freely in genetic decisions, most people are and will no doubt always be subject to the benevolent tyranny of expertise. Every expert knows how easy it is to get most people to choose one way rather than another simply by the way one raises the questions, describes the prognosis, and presents the options. The preferences of counselors will always overtly or subtly shape the choices of the counseled (Kass, 1999, p. 35).

Wertz and Fletcher share the same view:

> [I]t is extremely difficult, if not impossible for women to choose to reject technologies approved by the obstetrical profession. Once tests are offered, to reject them is a rejection of modern faith in science and also a rejection of modern beliefs that women should do everything possible for the health of the future child (Wertz & Fletcher, 1993, p. 175).

Often in genetics, it seems that clinicians and researchers believe that knowledge and genetic science are always and everywhere moral goods. This assumption is both seductive and infectious and left completely unscrutinised. The public believes that science and health care are founded upon altruism. They do not suspect or imagine how the power of science, or the power of expert knowledge, could potentially be used to harm them.

Clinicians use words which make it sound like the testing is good for everybody. The tests are 'to improve the prognosis' and 'to maximise the outcome for the baby' (Anderson, 1999, p. 129). They are made out to be all about protecting health – and who could reasonably say no to good health?

Given the level of trust and faith placed in medical professionals, it is not difficult to see why women would take their doctor's advice on abortion for foetal indications which were seen as negative – even if that meant a very late-term abortion. Studies show that large numbers of doctors support late abortions, even after 24 weeks for certain conditions.[21]

In Australia, a baby girl was aborted at 32 weeks for suspected dwarfism.[22] A subsequent survey showed 70 percent of obstetricians from around the country who specialise in ultrasound supported termination for dwarfism at 24 weeks (Toy, 2000).

Continuing a pregnancy with a baby likely to die before or soon after birth is considered pointless by many in the medical arena. There is an unquestioned assumption that it is better to abort than for a woman to deliver naturally – that her grief will be somehow lessened by ending the pregnancy quickly.[23]

But the women in this book challenge this widely held assumption. Teresa Streckfuss didn't think the births of Benedict and Charlotte were 'pointless'. Amy Kuebelbeck found meaning in the short life and natural death of her son.

Another grieving mother has written: 'We literally spent her entire lifetime holding her and loving her. I like thinking of it like that.'[24]

Rosemary Truman felt the same about her short-lived child. She wrote in *The Age*:

> We were able to hold her, bathe her, share our favourite places with her, show her off to our loved ones and special friends. She had a taste of life.
>
> It was the hardest and saddest time of our life. However, we learnt so much from this experience. I valued her life just as I have my other children. She gave us joy, pain, suffering, compassion, and love.
>
> It was worth every minute as I got to know her. To feel her beautiful spirit. She died in my arms and they will always feel empty without her.
>
> However, I know the joy of motherhood and I cherished every minute. I have a memory of her and I can keep that forever (Truman, 2001, p. 6).

And Nicolle Reece, the mother of Micah, wrote to me about her son:

> [So many people said] 'After all of that, and he just died anyway!' and 'It would have been so much easier if you had an abortion.' We are all going to 'die anyway'. Would you take your own life now because it will one day end? If you got a call today that your husband, sister, mother, friend . . . had just died, what would you give for one more hour? Two more hours? How about nine days? Easier for who? Easier for my husband and I? To face the rest of our life with guilt, doubt and 'what ifs' instead of love, hope and precious memories? . . . Easier for Micah? To be pulled from my body to die, without ever knowing the embraces, kisses and love of his family? (Reece, personal communication, 2003).

18

No assessment of the cost to women's health

Is anyone assessing the costs of these technologies to women's health and wellbeing? What does increasing genetic monitoring in pregnancy do for a woman's experience of pregnancy?

Barbara Katz Rothman illustrates how testing and the wait for results causes women not to announce or consider themselves even pregnant until the baby has passed the test (Rothman, 1986). She calls this the *tentative pregnancy*. Others have also explored how invasive eugenic-related checking can change the 'character and mood' of a pregnancy (Nolan, 1995, p. 499).

A 1998 *Lancet* study highlighted the present state of 'ignorance of the long-term psychological consequences of causing pregnant women to be anxious' (Boyd et al., 1998, p. 1581). A 2004 study on psychological effects of screening, referred to earlier, identified fifteen studies indicating that 'women do experience an acute response to receiving a screen-positive result'. Studies consistently reported women felt shock, panic, distress and worry upon receipt of a screen-positive test result. The anxiety caused changes to women's sleep patterns, appetite and feelings and attitudes about the pregnancy (Green et al., 2004, p. 27).

A Finnish study published in 1996 (Santalahti et al.) also reveals the negative emotions experienced by a significant number of women undergoing serum screening, amniocentesis and chorionic villus sampling:

> Thirty-three women (79%) described receiving a positive result as difficult and hard; several were frightened, shocked, or in panic. They experienced depression, distress, anxiety, and fear; their sleep was disturbed, and several cried . . . One woman – a health professional familiar with serum screening – described herself as 'out of control' (Santalahti et al., 1996, pp. 103–104).

The authors state that women who were waiting for results from amniocentesis or chorionic villous sampling (CVS) used the words 'hard, depressing, anxious, horrible, causing suffering, sad, and painful' to describe the time of waiting (Santalahti et al., 1996, p. 104).

The anxiety can persist even for women who are told their results are clear. Parents may ask 'If the baby doesn't have Down syndrome, what does it have?' (Green & Statham, 1996, p. 146). They experience 'lingering doubts produced by the belief that "there's no smoke without fire"' (Green & Statham, 1996, p. 154). An earlier study showed that three weeks after subsequent test results which overrode earlier indications of possible foetal abnormalities, women with a positive MSAFP were still more 'anxious and worried' about their baby's health, and 'held more negative attitudes toward their pregnancy', than the control group (in Santalahti et al., 1996, p. 102). In the Finnish study cited above, 18 per cent of the women surveyed remained worried about their baby's health even 10 weeks after normal amniocentesis or CVS results. One woman 'suspected that something abnormal was seen that was not revealed to her. She felt that something had happened to her: serum screening had struck her down' (Santalahti et al., 1996, p. 106).

This study's authors make the pertinent yet, in my view, under-explored observation that a woman's psychological state during pregnancy correlates with prenatal complications and with the future mother–child relationship. Negative experiences in pregnancy can also affect a mother's future wellbeing. The authors observe: 'The time of pregnancy is different from any other period in a woman's life, offering an opportunity for change and development. This positive possibility may be lost or lessened if the pregnancy is influenced by negative experiences' (Santalahti et al., 1996, p. 107).

Selective abortion for foetal impairment is counted as a gain in the health system and as a health benefit which seems to completely ignore the loss suffered by the parents. 'Counting a case prevented through termination of pregnancy as a success implies no value or a negative value to that life' (Hall et al., 1998, p. 757).

But where is there an assessment of the psychological and emotional costs of screening and subsequent abortion? Some studies indicate that abortion for suspected foetal abnormality places women at greater risk of post-abortion trauma.[25] A 1993 study found that 'women who terminate pregnancies for fetal anomalies experience grief as intense as those who experience spontaneous perinatal loss, and they may require similar clinical management' (Zeanah et al., 1993, p. 270). And what about the effects on women who almost aborted due to a false diagnosis? Some women have described how screening ruined their relationship with their child. Alison Brookes reports:

> One woman twice received a misdiagnosis of a neural tube defect in her fetus. After being subjected to the risk and emotional trauma of an unnecessary amniocentesis she found that her fetus (now her daughter) had no such problem. Relief at this late prognosis was not enough to undo the harm she believes this has done to her relationship with her child. As she was prepared to undergo a late termination if the results of the amniocentesis confirmed that her child would be affected, she spent nearly eight weeks of her pregnancy reconstructing her image of her fetus (Brookes, 1994, p. 3).

Tragically, the woman continues to feel guilty every time her daughter shows her any affection (Brookes, 1994, p. 3).

While prenatal screening has become common practice in many western countries, it is a different story in the Netherlands.

A 1996 law, the Population Screening Act, was instituted to protect the population against screening programs that could be a threat to the psychological and physical health of the person being screened. Ministerial approval is required for screening for 'serious disorders that can neither be treated nor prevented'. Termination of pregnancy is considered to be neither treatment nor prevention. It is against the law to offer prenatal screening to pregnant women unless they request it. Permission to offer prenatal diagnostic tests to pregnant women is given only if they are over 35 but the uptake of prenatal screening is relatively low. 'The question arises as to whether informed consent would be reduced if prenatal screening became routinised' (van den Berg et al., 2005, pp. 84–90).

Questions about risks of ultrasound and amniocentesis

Prenatal ultrasound has been identified as the most extensive prenatal diagnostic tool used without informed consent (Lippman, 1991, p. 21), yet a number of studies question assumptions that ultrasound is safe for women and their unborn children. All of the following have been identified in research: reduced foetal weight, a possible link with speech problems and damage to the central nervous system, the possibility of mutations, hereditable changes in DNA, and carcinogensis caused by high-frequency soundwaves used in ultrasound. The potential negative effects on women's ovaries caused by ultrasound energy are virtually ignored.[26]

Despite the lack of documented benefits from ultrasound, the practice has become so entrenched that it continues unquestioned and unabated. Even medical professionals who question the overuse of ultrasound and whether there is any real advantage to using it on pregnant women seem unwilling to cease, or even limit, its use.

Three members of staff of an obstetrics and gynaecology

department in Britain, commenting on a large prospective randomised trial on the effects of routine one-stage ultrasound screening in pregnancy, state that any 'theoretical advantage [of ultrasound screening] is not transferred to fetal or maternal outcome . . . Ultrasound screening failed to show any benefit in fetal weight or gestation at delivery.' However despite their critical views on the alleged benefits of ultrasound screening '[W]e continue ultrasound screening in our unit, despite its marginal benefits, and believe that mother and physician expect ultrasound as essential in the antenatal package' (Shafi et al., 1988, p. 804). Would women still expect or even want ultrasounds if some of the potential risks were made known to them, and the technology was not just served up without question?

The same mentality appears to apply to other types of testing. Doctors don't always believe that the tests they offer are clinically useful. A 1991 UK study revealed that many obstetricians routinely use tests they consider inaccurate (Ennis et al., 1991). A further 1994 study of obstetricians in England and Wales identified 35 percent as saying they were carrying out screening procedures because of outside pressures rather than because they considered them to be clinically valuable (Green, 1994).

Many women are also unaware of the risk of miscarriage after undergoing amniocentesis. A meta-analysis (Alfirevic et al., 2003) revealed that one in 125 pregnancies will be lost following the procedure. Another study showed that amniocentesis to check for Down syndrome caused up to four 'healthy babies' to be miscarried for every abnormality it detected (Leake & Milich, 2001). A recent study of 71,586 women (aged 35–49, with single births) in Sweden found that amniocentesis before 14 weeks gestation increased the risk of musculoskeletal postural deformities. Amniocentesis at 14 and 15 weeks increased the risk of respiratory disturbances. Subjecting women to clinically useless, inaccurate and risky tests has serious repercussions for their own and their babies' health (Cederholm et al., 2005).

Agonising decisions based on questionable findings

As stated earlier in this Introduction, many couples are having to make agonising decisions based on little or misleading information. The stories of a number of women in this book show how wrong the tests and/or their interpretation can be. There seems to be more concern in the medical profession about babies with non-normative conditions not being detected – slipping through the screening net – than about those aborted due to false diagnosis.

A six-year study, the results of which were published in *The Lancet* in 1998, found that 174 foetuses had a suspected abnormality identified on scan but *were subsequently found to be normal* [italics added]. *The Lancet* study found:

> Ultrasound soft markers lead to a small increase in detection of malformations but a large increase in false positives. Further research on the impact, including psychological, and value of markers is required to determine *whether the benefits of reporting them exceeds the harm* [italics added].
>
> There has been an increase in number of prenatal diagnoses of abnormality and a large increase in registration of suspicion of abnormality (ultrasound markers) with the baby appearing normal at birth (Boyd et al., 1998, pp. 1577, 1579).

The fear and sense of panic generated by suspicion of a condition following a scan can cause some couples to abort immediately, before follow-up testing. In two reported cases, termination was performed after suspicions raised by ultrasound scan of nuchal translucency in one baby and oesophageal atresia in the other. '[A]utopsy examination revealed normally formed fetuses' (Boyd et al., 1998, p. 1581).

A 2001 meta-analysis (Smith-Bindman et al., 2001, p. 1044), based on 56 studies between 1980 and 1999, urged clinicians to exercise caution about the use of ultrasound markers to advise women of their 'risk' of having a fetus with Down syndrome:

> . . . the overall sensitivity of this finding [thickened nuchal fold] is too low for it to be a practical screening test for Down syndrome . . . Using these markers as a basis for deciding to offer amnio-centesis will result in more fetal losses than cases of Down syndrome detected.

A 2000 study of 300 foetal autopsies found that the autopsy examination 'changed the prenatal "hypothesis" in 20 percent, provided extensive additional information in 41 percent and *confirmed the prenatal hypothesis in 39 percent*' [italics added] (Laussel-Riera et al., 2000). In other words, the prenatal diagnosis was only correct in 39 percent of cases. One wonders if the women whose babies were autopsied were told the results.

In 2003, a report in the *New Scientist* titled 'Test blunders risk needless abortions', found that errors in genetic tests for cystic fibrosis had prompted many US women to undergo risky foetal tests or abort a foetus that may have been healthy. In a commentary on this report, Kathy Hudson, Director of the Genetics and Public Policy Center in Washington D.C., wryly observed:

> In the US, there is more government oversight of the colouring used in M&Ms than there is for genetic tests that can have untold physical and emotional consequences, and the same is true in many other countries . . .
>
> We have our canary-in-the-mineshaft warning of the dangers of genetic screening. The physical and emotional stakes, not to

mention the legal implications, are too high to ignore it (Hudson, 2003, p. 5).

Another report tells the story of a woman who filed a lawsuit in 1998 because she aborted her four month old unborn child after an incorrect lab test. Janet Sheikhan, 42, contends that an amniocentesis performed in 1998 by the Lenox Hill Hospital, New York, and processed by a division of Genzyme Genetics showed that her unborn girl suffered from Edwards syndrome, a disease that causes mental retardation, after which she decided to have an abortion. She said that she later saw the pathology report on the child and it said there was no indication of the disease (CWNews.com. 1998).

Australian woman Kaylene Robson was 30 and pregnant with twin girls when, at 19 weeks, she was told that they were severely 'handicapped'. Her gynaecologist, on examining the ultrasound results, told her that one twin had spina bifida and no skull, and the other was missing major organs and three chambers in her heart. He said the twins also suffered twin-to-twin transfusion and told her to abort. 'He said the babies had to go because they were so deformed with abnormalities that there was no hope of them surviving . . . He said they were going to die inside me anyway, so they had to go' Ms Robson said. Against her gynaecologist's advice, she obtained a second opinion and the babies were later born – with none of the conditions originally diagnosed (Lambert, 1996b, p. 37).

Another account comes from California, USA, about a baby who proved wrong the doctors who had pressured her parents to abort her – even at nine months' gestation (Ball, 2003). Doctors twice advised Kimberley Frazier, 20, to abort her pregnancy. The first time was at five-and-a-half months when the baby's heart defect was first identified and Frazier developed a kidney infection, and again at nine months when doctors told her the baby was unlikely to survive delivery. The baby did survive, and Frazier and her partner were 'bitter about the advice to abort.'

David Magnus, co-director of the Center for Bio-Medical Ethics at Stanford University, was quoted as saying that recommending termination was not unreasonable and that abortion could 'protect the parents of the fetus from further emotional pain' – as though there were no emotional pain involved in the abortion of a child, especially late in the pregnancy (see Tankard Reist, 2000).

In 1996, Denise McCarthy was told by doctors in Sydney, Australia, that her child had either Down syndrome or cystic fibrosis. She refused to terminate and Grace was born perfectly healthy (Lambert, 1996a). However, Ms McCarthy didn't receive much sympathy for the unnecessary anxiety she went through because of the false indications. Melbourne ultrasound specialist Dr Lachlan de Crespigny appeared more concerned about the babies who weren't caught by the screening. He stated that diagnosing abnormalities that did not exist was *less of a problem* than failing to detect abnormalities. 'A number of spina bifida cases are being missed in this country and that is a real concern for us,' he said (in Lambert, 1996a, p. 7).[27]

Lack of knowledge among medical professionals

Not only are the results of screening often questionable, so is the level of knowledge among health professionals about the conditions they think they have detected. The authors of a 2001 study reported in the *British Medical Journal* identified as their main finding the

> . . . enormous variation between different health professionals in what they knew, thought, and told parents . . .
>
> It is disturbing to note the haphazard nature of how parents were informed of the diagnosis, what information was given, and what was implied . . . there were . . . examples of grossly inadequate

or frankly misleading information being given (Abramsky et al., 2001, p. 466).[28]

A father is quoted as saying:

> The consultant appeared to know little about the condition, but seemed to expect us to make a judgement based on the fact that an abnormal result had occurred. I am glad that we insisted on finding out more about the condition before we were willing to make our decision, otherwise we could have decided to terminate through ignorance alone – instead we now have a lovely son (in Abramsky et al., 2001, p. 465).

Voicing similar sentiments, a mother said:

> In retrospect, I feel rather shocked that parents in our situation should have so routinely been offered the option of termination – particularly without first being offered appropriate counselling . . . [I] felt that research papers we were shown at the hospital were both outdated and one sided (in Abramsky et al., 2001, p. 465).

Yet another woman commented how upset she was by the information she was initially given and the way it was given:

> The result of the amniocentesis was given over the telephone followed by some outdated information. I felt distraught when I first received the result – however the geneticist assured me that my baby would be perfectly normal, and she is! The initial information intimated that she could be severely retarded. Some people may have terminated at this stage without expert advice. This horrifies me (in Abramsky et al., 2001, p. 465).

The ignorance of too many in the medical professional must be urgently addressed.

'They turn the baby into a monster!':
Lack of information on disability and support

Not only is the information that is provided often slanted in a way to encourage termination – even when the indications on which such recommendations are based are questionable. Parents are generally not given information or directed to groups which would help them better understand particular disabilities and are thus less able to see how the child may fare and the support that is available. It seems they are often provided with the worst possible scenarios about particular disabilities, and the information they are given is skewed one way. For example, Lisa Blumberg observes:

> Emphasis may be placed in genetic counselling on the difficulties a condition may produce, but not on how people cope with these difficulties.
>
> ... Parents may be given illustrated medical abstracts but rarely are they given copies of *Exceptional Parent* and *Disability Rag*. They may have been told as they are in 'A Time to Decide, A Time to Heal', a booklet prepared by a genetic counsellor at Michigan State University, that 'one benefit that may be attributed to [pregnancy] interruption is the prevention of the child's mental and physical suffering.' However, they are not exposed to views such as those of disability activists Michelle Fine and Adrienne Asch that, the 'pain and "tragedy" of living with a disability in our culture derives primarily from the pain and humiliation of discrimination, oppression and anti-disability attitudes, not from the disability,' nor are they usually told of how disabled and non-disabled people are working with some considerable success to change society (Blumberg, 1994b, p. 143).

A potent example of 'one-sided negative information' provided to women is given in an excellent article on the malfunction of informed consent in prenatal diagnostic programs. A transcript of a telephone conversation between a genetic counsellor and a telephone volunteer with a retinal cancer foundation shows how the counsellor wants statistics, and the volunteer, who has retinal cancer, wants to offer help and support to the patient the counsellor represents. The volunteer points out that the counsellor is being directive, by presenting his patient 'with merely clinical data' rather than connecting her with those who have the condition and are enjoying life.[29]

In the Australian study on prenatal screening by Alison Brookes, 'Vivienne' also decries this lack of information:

> They should give them the option to talk to somebody who has [a child with a genetic condition]. You get pressured into getting rid of it instead of [a choice]. They only ever tell you how bad it is going to be. You don't get the choice of talking to someone who's got a disabled child (in Brookes, 1998, p. 210).

'Brenda' – also in Brookes' study – reports similar feelings. It was only because she'd cared for a child with a genetic condition that she withstood negative predictions by her doctors for a later child. As she put it:

> [Without this experience] I possibly would have had an abortion because of the fear of not knowing. And I do really believe that the doctors always present with the worst-case scenario . . . and fear, just fear and not knowing what the baby possibly could have been. I think I probably would have had an abortion. Which would have been really, really difficult, something that would have been very hard for me to live with. If they're going to present that side, then they've also got to present the side of this really cute little kid, you know? So, they might be a handful, but there are a lot of kids who are a handful. I think they should present the information to the parents on a more 50-50 basis and not all 'This is terrible, this is what you're in for' (in Brookes, 2001, p. 141).

As 'Brenda' states succinctly: 'They turn the baby into a monster!' (in Brookes, 1998, p. 210).

Chris Nugent wrote to me about her daughter, Grace, who had been diagnosed at about 19 weeks with trisomy 18. She had asked for information and support – but it never came. 'In this day of "choice" the medical community did not support our choice to continue,' she wrote (Chris Nugent, personal communication, 31 May, 2004).

> The counsellor emphasised how horrible and fatal this condition was. We told her that termination was not an option for us. We got the response 'Are you doing this for religious reasons?' They did not know what to do with a couple who decided to continue a pregnancy like this in spite of the diagnosis. I asked her if she had any support for me. She said she would get back to me and give me the name of someone who had a child like this. I am still waiting ... She said there was a lot of support if we terminated, she offered us nothing to continue with the pregnancy. I was shocked. The doctors and medical people at the big hospital didn't get us. My baby and I were under attack. Their goal was to have us terminate before 24 weeks. They did not give us an ounce of hope or support.

If this imbalance was redressed, and the option of having a child with a disability allowed to be considered and explored, more couples would be likely to choose to continue the pregnancy, as the following suggests. Of the 55 couples who contacted the Down Syndrome Adoption Exchange, USA, in 1990 after prenatal diagnosis, only two decided to place their child for adoption and *none* opted for abortion.[30] This needs to be contrasted with the case of a British doctor who starved to death a baby girl who had Down syndrome. He was acquitted because the judge found it was ethical that a child with Down syndrome should not survive.[31]

Women can be a lot more resilient than they are given credit for. Sometimes those around them are more upset than they are. 'Eliza', in Brookes' study, remembers:

> When I found out I felt all right about it, I mean I didn't feel happy that my son would have to go through life like this, but I felt at least he's going to be alive. I can cope with that much. And whatever comes along, we'll just deal with it as it comes along. My friends' reactions were like how awful, how must you feel, and I felt like, I almost felt guilty because I thought I should be more upset about it than I was. People just kept expecting that this week I may not collapse over it, but next week I probably will. And, I never have gone to that end of the earth, you know. There have been times that I have not coped, but most of the time I do. People just thought that was the end of my life, and it's not! (in Brookes, 1998, p. 220).

One genetic counsellor, Barbara Biesecker, says it should not be assumed that an initial grief reaction means a woman does not want to continue the pregnancy. She may just need a chance to readjust her expectations (as the author of 'Welcome to Holland', a fable quoted in Julia Anderson's story in this book, did). In an editorial in the *British Medical Journal*, Biesecker writes:

> Patients suffer a loss when they receive a prenatal diagnosis about their foetus. The loss is often not of the foetus that comes to carry the diagnosis but of the foetus the parents hoped they carried. This grief is profound yet does not preclude a woman's ability to welcome an affected foetus into the world. Others, including health care providers, may interpret this grief as rejection of the affected foetus. Women have been articulate about their resentment of such assumptions. Often the grief represents a readjustment of expectations, and women who experience this loss appreciate those who accept it as part of adjustment and do

not conclude from it unwillingness to continue the pregnancy (Biesecker, 2001, p. 441).

Too often, however, rather than being given time to adjust, to learn more about their child's condition and explore support services, parents are immediately scheduled for an abortion.

Dehumanising and stigmatising labels

Most women cannot dismiss their unborn children – no matter their imperfections – as easily as some in the medical profession seem able to do. It seems the weight and meaning women give their babies count for little to those who prefer to bring into the world what they think of as 'unproblematic people' (Rowland, 1992, p. 81). The belief that allowing these children to be born would bring misery into the world and that they would have second-rate lives leads to a depersonalising and devaluing of the worth of any child whatever his or her abilities.

If we accept the criteria often used to justify terminating the lives of babies with disabilities, that they will lead 'a horrible life', full of 'pain and suffering', then we may also have to acquiesce to the selection and elimination of any children who may be born into harsh circumstances, for example baby girls in countries where they are also likely to 'lead a horrible life' and suffer great hardship. Some already see this as justification for selection and abortion. Sakuntala Narasimban, writing in *The New Internationalist*, cites the Indian custom, 'Better to snuff a life at birth than to suffer lifelong misery,' and quotes a local female medical doctor as agreeing with it. 'These mothers have suffered so much, they don't want the pattern repeated in their own lives' (Narasimban, 1993, p. 240).

Of course, it is girl children who are very often considered defective and genetically deficient. As Brock L. Eide comments:

> Such criteria ['horrible life'] could also be used to justify abortion
> for sex selection – a practice almost universally condemned by

Western bioethicists – especially in countries such as India and China where there are clear differences in expected quality of life for male and female children, and where females can be highly restricted in their ability to form and fulfil their own sets of values. *Indeed, such subjective third-party assessments of quality of life are unavoidably elastic, capable of being stretched to accommodate whatever concerns or biases the assessor may have* [italics added]. Such considerations should give us pause, and lead us to wonder whether Leon Kass was perhaps right in claiming that the principle '"Defectives" should not be born' is a principle without limits (Eide, 1997, p. 61).

Some disability activists have drawn parallels with the way the disabled unborn child is described and the way they themselves are viewed.

Language reinforces the negativity. Terms like 'fetal deformity' and 'defective fetus' are deeply stigmatizing, carrying connotations of inadequacy and shame. Many of us have been called 'abnormal' by medical personnel, who view us primarily as 'patients', subject to the definitions and control of the medical profession (Hershey, 1994, p. 29).

Lisa Blumberg argues that the term 'defective fetus' should be seen to be in the same category as 'kike fetus' and 'nigger fetus' (Blumberg, 1994b, p. 153). Anne Godfrey of Queensland, Australia, told me (personal communication, 16 March, 2004) that when her unborn child was diagnosed with Down syndrome four years ago, the doctor told her, 'It'll only be a pet.'[32]

It needs to be pointed out that many nurses are also unable to depersonalise the foetus in the way they are expected to. Elisabeth Boetzkes records the following disturbing account in an article about genetic terminations:

[O]ne nurse told of contacting a physician for advice the first time she delivered a live baby. (This is rare, but when it happens, babies may breathe on their own for five to twenty minutes). The physician simply told her to 'drop it into the saline solution.' Ethically this was not an option for her. She said, 'These babies are human beings that deserve to be treated with dignity and caring.' What she did was clean and dress the baby and carry him around with her until he stopped breathing. She then took him to his parents (Boetzkes et al., 2002, p. 126).[33]

Natalie Withers, quoted earlier, is pained that the doctors recorded her daughter's age at one day less than 20 weeks to avoid a death certificate. Natalie feels this undermines the humanity of her daughter. 'People don't consider them to be a person. It insults me still to this day. I think it's a societal thing – because she's disabled, she doesn't count,' she says (personal communication, 13 May, 2005).

Chris Nugent (2004) felt her child was being depersonalised by those who thought she should abort.

We just had a perfect baby and now you are telling me she is a 'fetus with a fatal defect.' What the hell does that mean? Our baby was no longer our baby, instead in the medical community she became a 'fetus with a defect.' We said that termination was not an option for us. They [medical personnel] looked at us like we were from another planet . . . Grace Anne was born July 26, 2002 by elective c-section. She lived for 62 days and died September 26, 2002. We got much more than we ever dreamed . . . I didn't see trisomy 18, I just saw my precious little girl. That is what most people realised when she was born. She wasn't the monster the doctors had painted for me four months before – she was just a little sweetheart. All she needed was love. Boy, did she get it!

But there are some who don't think babies – and adults – with conditions like this should get any love at all. Attorney Jason Brent and Jon Evans, writing in *Lament*, the newsletter of the Los Angeles chapter of Mensa ('the exclusive club for people with IQ in the top two percent'), have argued that people with physical and mental disabilities are mere 'pieces of meat' and that society must face up to the need to 'kill off the old, the weak, the stupid and the inefficient (in Zamichow, 1995, p. B1).'[34]

The rise of eugenicist thought

Where do these attitudes come from – these views that those with unacceptably low IQ (Rifkin, 1998, p. 155), the genetically unworthy, the physically and mentally – and racially – imperfect should not be permitted to breathe the same air as everyone else? They have a long history whose lessons have not been entirely learnt. The history of what is sometimes identified as the 'old' eugenics is instructive in any examination of the new genetics and genetic screening. While I acknowledge that eugenic thought goes back at least to Plato, I limit this brief overview to eugenics over the last hundred years.[35]

The Racial Hygiene Society was formed in Germany in 1905, the English Eugenics Education Society in 1907, the American Eugenics Society in 1923, while eugenic ideas advanced in non-English-speaking countries as divergent as Norway, Brazil and the Soviet Union (Buchanan et al., 2000, p. 31). The Racial Hygiene Association, formed in Australia in the 1920s, reminded women that motherhood was 'not an instinct but a science' (Galton, 2001).

In a recent book remarkable for its detail, *War against the weak: Eugenics and America's campaign to create a master race*, Edwin Black documents the efforts of those who 'would hunt, identify, label and take control of those deemed unfit to populate the earth' (Black, 2003, p. 87). He quotes Harry Laughlin, Director of the

Eugenics Record Office and a witness in the Carrie Buck sterilisation case: 'To purify the breeding stock of the race at all costs is the slogan of eugenics.' Laughlin's three-pronged program was based on compulsory sterilisation, mass incarceration, and sweeping immigration restrictions.[36]

John D. Rockefeller shared Laughlin's views. Black describes how

[O]n January 27, 1912, using his personal 26 Broadway stationery (John D.) Rockefeller wrote [of his] plan to incarcerate feeble-minded criminal women for an extra length of time, so they 'would . . . be kept from perpetuating [their] kind . . . until after the period of child bearing had passed' (Black, 2003, p. 93).

Black gives a frightening account of the enactment of sterilisation laws in the US, best known through the story of their first victim, Carrie Buck.[37] On 10 September 1924, a colony review board ruled that Carrie Buck was 'feebleminded and by the laws of heredity is the probable potential parent of socially inadequate offspring, likewise afflicted . . .' and as such, 'she may be sexually sterilized . . . and that her welfare and that of society will be promoted by her sterilization . . .' (in Black, 2003, pp. 113–114). Justice Holmes of the United States Supreme Court, referring to Carrie's mother, Carrie and her daughter Vivien, famously declared that 'three generations of imbeciles are enough.' He said:

. . . it would be strange if it [the state] could not call upon those who already sap the strength of the state for these lesser sacrifices, often not felt to be such by those concerned, in order to prevent our being swamped with incompetence . . . It is better for all the world, if instead of waiting to execute degenerate offspring for crime, or to let them starve for their imbecility, society can prevent those who are manifestly unfit from continuing their kind. The principle that sustains compulsory vaccination is broad enough to cover cutting the Fallopian tubes (in Black, 2003, p. 121).

It was somewhat ironic that Carrie's 'socially inadequate offspring', Vivien, was to be adopted by J. T. Dobbs, a Charlottsville peace officer.[38] Vivien went on to perform well educationally – she was described as 'above average' and her name listed on an honour roll – despite Justice Holmes having classified her an imbecile.[39]

The sterilisation crusade went ahead in leaps and bounds, fired up by the Buck ruling. And as if it wasn't enough to be sterilised against your will, you were also expected to pay for it. 'If the patient or his family is financially able to reimburse the state it is required to do so.' The price for the loss of the right to reproduce was fifty dollars (in Trombley, 1988, p. 66).

An example of the 'process' by which a sterilisation determination was reached is provided in the following extracts from hospital records in the 1940s involving a Mrs W. who was sterilised in 1942 aged sixteen (in Trombley, 1988, pp. 242–243).

(Lynchburg, June 3, 1942) [40]

Q. You don't object to this operation, do you?

A. Well, it's no use to.

Q. Why do you say, 'It's no use to'?

A. Because I know I am going to be operated on anyway.

Mrs W. was brought before the board again on 5 August 1942.

Mr . . . Have you th[ ] [ ] matter any since the last time you were here?

Mrs W: Well, I still don't want to be, but I am not going to [ ] some of the girls and some of the attendants have talked to me and [ ] better now than I did.

Q. You do? Well I am glad you have come to the conclusion [sic]. We [ ] interested in punishing you in any way. We simply believe that [ ] if and have a feeble-minded or [ ] epileptic child instead of that child [ ] pleasure to you, she would be – it would be a constant sorrow all [ ] and all of her life; that's the only reason we want to sterilize you [ ] young and attractive and the chances are that if you live you may [ ] who will want to marry you and set up a home. That's a wholly desi[ ] [ ] natural thing. The world is established on homes. We believe that [ ] child in your arms who was like one of these unfortunates here, it [ ] source of pleasure and comfort to you at all. It wouldn't be that [ ] it wouldn't. That's all we want of you: I am glad you came to that [ ]

Mrs W. had been convinced by staff and other inmates at the home that unless she 'consented' to sterilisation, she would never get out of the home at Lynchburg (Trombley, 1988, p. 243).[41]

Resistance of clients and relatives was identified as 'a major problem'. Their reluctance was put down to their inability to see beyond themselves. Women who regretted the operation were labelled 'maladjusted'. 'Where unfavourable results were observed, they were associated with neurotic personality and maladjustment in the life situation' (Trombley, 1988, p. 170).[42]

Birth control and eugenics

The pioneers of the birth control movement, Margaret Sanger and Marie Stopes, were passionate about their eugenic convictions.[43] Sanger's slogan was 'more children from the fit, less from the unfit – that is the chief issue in Birth Control' (in Black, 2003, p. 131).

Sanger was in favour of mass sterilisation of those deemed defective, large-scale incarceration of those judged unfit, and harsh immigration restrictions. In Sanger's view, the lower classes and the unfit were 'human waste' not worth helping. She quoted freely the extreme eugenic view that human 'weeds' should be 'exterminated'.[44] (Vilification of groups and individuals is, of course, a well-known precursor to the withdrawal of their rights.)[45]

Every feeble-minded girl or woman of the hereditary type, especially of the *moron class* [emphasis added], should be segregated during the reproductive period . . . Moreover, when we realise that each feeble-minded person is a potential source of an endless progeny of defect, we prefer the policy of immediate sterilisation, of making sure that parenthood is absolutely prohibited to the feeble-minded (Margaret Sanger quoted in Black, 2003, p. 131).

Marie Stopes didn't have much patience for 'morons' either. In 1924, after finding in her mail a letter from the deaf father of deaf children, Stopes wrote to the superintendent of the school the father had attended:

I should be much obliged if you would tell me how it came about that two persons educated at [the Royal Association in Aid of the Deaf and Dumb] were permitted to marry and bring forth children, all of whom are still more imperfect and a burden on the country . . . Do you think it advisable that two defectives, both brought up at public expense, should be permitted to produce four defectives to be brought up at public expense and where is this geometrical progression going to stop? (in Greer, 1984, p. 309).[46]

It wasn't only strangers who incited Stopes to fury. Her own son was the victim of her wrath when he ignored his mother's wishes and married Mary Barnes Wallis. Stopes refused to recognise her daughter-in-law. Why was she so venomous towards her? Because Ms Wallis wore glasses. Marie Stopes put it bluntly:

The essential is health in a potential mother and she has an inherited disease of the eyes which not only makes her wear hideous glasses so that it is horrid to look at her, but the awful curse will carry on and I have the horror of our line being so contaminated and little children with the misery of glasses . . . Mary and Harry are quite callous about both the wrong to their children, the wrong to my family and the eugenic crime (1949, in Greer, 1984, p. 310).

The marriage went ahead, Marie Stopes did not attend and her son was cut out of his mother's will (Trombley, 1988, p. 81).

Eugenics and extermination

The American eugenists were big fans of Hitler's plans for a racially pure Germany. This is demonstrated in the 1932 March–April edition of *Eugenical News*: 'The Aryans are the great founders of civilisations . . . The mixing of blood, the pollution of race . . . has been the sole reason why old civilisations have died out.' A 1934 issue stated: 'But may we be the first to thank this one man, Adolf Hitler, and to follow him on the way towards a biological salvation of humanity' (in Black, 2003, p. 305).

Like other moves internationally to limit the numbers of those deemed unfit, Hitler's also began with sterilisation. It appears he got the idea from America in the first place – something of which the American eugenicists were very proud. To them, America's sterilisation program could not be faulted. *Eugenical News* also claimed that in the 16,000 sterilisations performed in America over recent years, not a single 'eugenical mistake' had been made (in Black, 2003, p. 301).

Germany's Law for the Prevention of Defective Progeny was decreed on 14 July 1933. It required mass compulsory sterilisation. The Reich determined that 400,000 Germans would undergo the procedure from 1 January 1934 and that doctors who failed to report their suspect patients would be fined (Black, 2003, pp. 299, 300).

But sterilisation was not enough for Germany to be rid of its useless eaters. The next step was euthanasia. Starting from 1940, thousands of Germans were taken from old age homes, mental institutions and other facilities and systematically gassed. Between

50,000 and 100,000 were eventually killed (Black, 2003, p. 317). It is estimated that between 200,000 and 250,000 mentally and physically disabled people were murdered from 1939 to 1945 under the Operation T4 and other 'euthanasia' programs.[47] After this, it was a 'short hop from euthanasia to genocide' (Rothblatt, 1997, p. 62).

Elizabeth R. Schiltz has written a profoundly affecting essay, reprinted in this book, drawing parallels between the Nazi mentality and the current medical thinking which would have de-selected her much-loved son before he was born.

Daniel Kevles concludes his history of the eugenics movement:

> . . . eugenics has proved itself historically to have been often a cruel and always a problematic faith, not least because it has elevated abstractions – the 'race,' the 'population,' and more recently the 'gene pool' – above the rights and needs of individuals and their families (Kevles, 1985, pp. 300–301).

The new 'nice' eugenics

While many in the scientific establishment don't want to admit it, much of what masquerades as purely health, reassurance and beneficent reasons for screening is actually underpinned by a eugenic philosophy which has as its core a belief that says there is an *unacceptable way of being human* (Hauerwaus in Reinders, 2000).

Tucker Carlson, in a 1996 article in *The Weekly Standard* titled 'Eugenics, American style: The abortion of Down syndrome babies', quotes a physician who refuses to use the word eugenics: 'Sometime you need to abandon words that have common meanings that connote the wrong ethics or morals.' Carlson adds, 'But only the words have changed' (in Buchanan et al., 2000, p. 55). Abby Lippman concurs:

Though the word 'eugenics' is scrupulously avoided in most bio-medical reports about prenatal diagnosis, except where it is strongly disclaimed as a motive for intervention, this is disingenuous. Prenatal diagnosis presupposes that certain fetal conditions are intrinsically not bearable (Lippman, 1991, pp. 24–25).

And Jeremy Rifkin points out that the many new scientific discoveries and inventions 'now make possible the kind of eugenic society that earlier eugenics reformers only could have dreamed of achieving' (Rifkin, 1998, p. 117).

'Preventing the existence of people with disabilities' and 'Why we are morally obliged to genetically enhance our children' were the titles of two papers delivered at a conference on Ethics, Science and Moral Philosophy of Assisted Human Reproduction at the Royal Society, London in September 2004.

While most supporters of large scale genetic screening go to great lengths to be seen as opposed to the odious practices of eugenicists of the past (so as not to arouse our suspicions?), others are more forthcoming. In 1971, the geneticist Bentley Glass proclaimed: 'No parents will in that future time have a right to burden society with a malformed or a mentally incompetent child' (in Kass, 1999, p. 35). In 2003, John Harris, a bioethicist at Manchester University, told the BBC that eugenics was a laudable aim. 'Eugenics is the attempt to create fine healthy children and that's everyone's ambition.' Couples who choose to have disabled babies were 'misguided', he said (in Australasian Bioethics Information, 2003).

'Misguided' is too soft a word for some. Test-tube baby pioneer and an expert on pre-implantation diagnosis, Robert Edwards has been quoted as saying: 'Soon it will be a sin of parents to have a child that carries the heavy burden of genetic disease. We are entering a world where we have to consider the quality of our children' (in Griffiths, 1999).

43

China is quite upfront about its eugenic aims. In 1994 it introduced the Maternal and Infant Health Care Law which uses pre-marital check-ups, marriage bans, sterilisation and abortion to 'improve the quality of the newborn population'. Under Articles 10 and 16, there can be no legal challenge to a physician's order for sterilisation or termination of pregnancy. The bill was originally named 'On Eugenics and Health Protection', and used phrases such as 'inferior births'. It was renamed following an international outcry, but the intent of the law did not change. Beijing professor Xiao Fei defended the law by saying: 'If we can limit the number of these people [with disabilities] the country will shed some of its burden' (in Post, 1994, p. 74).

Lawyer and geneticist Margery Shaw is also into the shedding of 'burdens'. In her view, abortion for foetal abnormality is morally obligatory and she has called for legal penalties against parents who ignore their moral duties and give birth to babies with disabilities. Parents who knowingly give birth to a seriously impaired child, she says, are guilty of negligent child abuse. Shaw (1980) wants courts and legislatures to hold parents accountable for the genetic health of their children. Shaw (1984) says those who have disabled children should be put in reproductive 'quarantine' because '[s]ociety cannot allow parents to have "defective" children' (in Blumberg, 1994, p. 146).

This is where the echoes from a previous age become louder. Shaw's 'reproductive quarantine' resonates with the decree of American pioneer eugenicist Laughlin in 1914 that the mothers of unfit children should be relegated to 'a place comparable to that of the females of mongrel strains of domestic animals' (in Black, 2003, p. 89).

Like Shaw, Eric Rakowski also believes parents need to be held accountable for their choices. Those who 'chose to bear genetically disadvantaged children when they might have non-disadvantaged' ones, should incur greater insurance liability because 'they could not fairly push the cost of their choices off on other members of the insurance pool' (Rakowski, 2002, p. 1345). They also become candidates for 'coerced contraception'.[48]

Insurers or government officials, Rakowski continues, 'might find it worthwhile to *encourage* [italics added] pregnant women to run some surgical risks [in utero surgery] or to abort and try again, by providing medical care, counselling, or other types of support free of charge' (Rakowski, 2002, p. 1392).

The provision of what would clearly be directive counselling aimed at securing an abortion outcome is seen by Rakowski as entirely legitimate. One wonders what becomes of his generous provision of medical care, counselling and support if the pregnant woman does not accept the 'encouragement' he recommends.

Testing and termination as a bargain: 'Units of handicapped prevented'

Of course, all these technologies are underpinned by a cost-benefit analysis in which the abortion of a baby with a disability becomes just an economic transaction. Kass has identified an 'upsurge of economic pressures to limit reproductive freedom . . .' (1999, p. 35).

Australian geneticist, Professor Grant Sutherland, has said, 'if you prevent the birth of a child with Down's syndrome you are probably saving the community a million dollars or more in the life of the child'. The Human Genetics Society of Australasia, of which Professor Sutherland was the immediate past president, had urged governments in 1992 to set up centralised public clinics to provide structured screening of pregnant women using a new Down syndrome test. Professor Sutherland said the new approach would be cost-effective if it prevented just a few cases of Down syndrome each year, as each 'sufferer' put an enormous drain on community resources because of special needs (in *Adelaide Advertiser*, 1992, p. 16).

Harris et al., writing in *The Lancet*, justify the cost of particular screening because the results of several studies suggested '. . . the costs of offering amniocentesis would be offset by the savings associated with preventing the birth of an infant affected by Down's syndrome' (2004, pp. 276–282).[49]

Economic imperatives drive the way the debate on prenatal diagnosis is framed. Angus Clarke, also writing in *The Lancet*, has observed:

> An unacceptable measure of outcome audit, for example, would be utilisation of population-based data (e.g. numbers of terminations for a specified condition or a trend in birth incidence). If a department's work is to be measured in such terms, there will be subtle – and possibly less than subtle – pressure upon clinicians to maximise the rate of termination of pregnancy for 'costly' disorders . . . To some extent, clinical geneticists have brought this risk upon themselves by seeking to justify their continued financial support in terms of cost-benefit analysis . . . Clinical geneticists must now disengage their profession from its self-justification in such terms, rather than to continue to employ the eugenic vocabulary of social responsibility in reproduction . . .
>
> It is not at all far-fetched to imagine finance for the care of the handicapped being reduced on the grounds that there will be fewer handicapped children in the genetics services operated more 'efficiently.' To encourage such services to meet targets in terms of termination, our funding might depend upon 'units of handicapped prevented' which would pressurise parents into screening programs and then into unwanted terminations with the active collusion of clinical geneticists anxious about their budgets (Clarke, 1990, pp. 1146–1147).[50]

Tom Shakespeare, in his 'Manifesto for Genetic Justice', writes of 'a pernicious tendency to develop screening policies on the grounds of cost-benefit models':

> These arguments balance the cost of detecting and terminating affected pregnancies with the cost of supporting a disabled person throughout their life. Particular policies are defended in terms of a reduction to the welfare or medical bills of a nation. This rests on highly dubious assumptions about the cost of being disabled. It replaces human rights with economic rationality. It ignores the fact that anybody could become impaired at any time due to accidents or disease, not just the very small number of people who are born with impairment (Shakespeare, 1999, p. 31).

The quest for perfection and the gospel of gene salvation

Driving the international genetic screening push is not only cost, but a philosophical view of the notion of perfection. The desire for perfect bodies – the cult of bodily perfection and obsession with image – is reflected in dangerous dieting, weight loss regimes and cosmetic surgery. Modelling agencies report that increasing numbers of younger women are having breast surgery. In China, young women subject themselves to torturous procedures in which steel rods are screwed into their legs to try to gain a few extra centimetres in height.[51] The desire for perfect bodies extends to a desire for perfect foetuses, which also means a desire for perfect eggs and sperm.

Ethicist Daniel Callahan observes:

> Behind the human horror at genetic defectiveness lurks . . . an image of the perfect human being. The very language of 'defect', 'abnormality', 'disease', and 'risk' presupposes such an image, a kind of proto-type of perfection (in Peter, 1971, p. 1133).

In a 2002 lecture, the famous geneticist James Watson spoke of the need to eradicate 'undesirable traits' in children through genetic engineering. 'Who wants an ugly baby?' he asked. 'Going for perfection was something I always thought you should do' (in Abraham, 2002, p. A1). The 'father' of DNA science, Watson has called for laws to be changed so that scientists could alter the genes of sperm, eggs and embryos and so 'rid genetic defects from future generations' (in Conor, 2001).

Australian ethicist Julian Savulescu, now Uehiro Chair in Practical Ethics at the University of Oxford, believes it far preferable for people to use reproductive technologies to have genetically unrelated children if having a biologically related child would result in an inferior product. 'If medicine has an absolute commitment to maximization, doctors should only offer to bring into existence those individuals who are expected . . . to have the best lives' (Savulescu, 1999, p. 19).[52]

The quest for perfection continues through new advances in genetic engineering enabling the alteration of sperm, eggs and embryos (germ-line therapy) or altering genes in children (somatic cell therapy) (Stock, 2002). Such feats have been dreamt of for years. In his book *On human nature*, E. O. Wilson (1978, p. 208) reflected that genetic enhancement techniques might mean the following:

> New patterns of sociality could be installed in bits and pieces. It might be possible to imitate genetically the more nearly perfect nuclear family of the white-handed gibbon or the harmonious sisterhoods of the honeybees.

Gregory Stock, in *Redesigning humans*, believes that freedom to choose includes freedom to enhance our progeny even by inserting animal DNA into human embryos,[53] inserting or removing chromosomes, inserting artificial chromosomes into a genetically engineered embryo, or altering human capacities through nanotechnology. Stock believes the desire for tailor-made children with 'the most up-to-date chromosome enhancements' will become so ingrained that parents won't see laboratory conception as burdensome (Stock, 2002, p. 185).

Bioethicists John A. Robertson and Jean E. Chambers extend an absolute right to abortion to an entitlement to use technology in order to choose the genetic makeup of a child and create 'quality control offspring'. Chambers argues that having a child is a major investment and it's imperative to get it right. '[T]he candidate embryos are effectively at the woman's disposal,' she says (in Smith, 2004, p.145). Gregory Pence, in *Who's afraid of human cloning?*, argues that if we think it is important to match the breed of dogs to the needs of owners, parents should be allowed to match a child to their needs using cloning.[54] In Pence's view, parents are 'obligated' to genetically enhance their offspring. 'It is wrong to choose lives for future people that make them much worse off than they otherwise could have been' (Pence, 1998, p. 114). This provides another example of the way in which children are increasingly viewed as 'commodities'. As such, they can be improved upon, bought, sold, traded and used for spare parts.[55]

Ethicists like Australian Peter Singer, now a professor at Princeton University, have helped feed a view that we should be creating the 'best' children possible by genetically engineering them from the embryo stage. Singer has called for government subsidies to parents to 'genetically improve their offspring' (Kuhse & Singer, 1985). This is the same Peter Singer who advocates the killing of disabled newborns.[56]

In an address to the Murdoch Children's Research Institute in 2000 titled 'Shopping at the genetic supermarket', Singer predicted we would be able to insert genetic material into embryos within twenty years. Once a few parents started using the practice, others would feel obliged to follow suit. 'Even if a minority of parents used genetic engineering initially, other parents would be under pressure to ensure their children were not disadvantaged relative to their peers,' Peter Singer said (in Button, 2000, p. 3).

On the Australian Broadcasting Corporation's *7.30 Report* the next day, ethicist Nicholas Tonti-Filippini criticised the 'grand supermarket' idea:

> The grand supermarket, it won't be a supermarket selling disabled children or different children or children who are dwarfs. It will be a supermarket of the supposedly highly intelligent, those with great characteristics – tallness, physical prowess and so on – and so suddenly we'll be valuing people for those things rather than just valuing them because they're people (ABC, 2000, August 23).

There is no room for imperfect individuals in the world of the Transhumanist movement either. Founded in 1998, the World Transhumanist Association devotes itself to promoting the rights of people to redesign themselves and their children so as to have 'better minds, better bodies and better lives' and to be 'better than well' (Hughes, n.d.).[57]

If the attitudes expressed here make most people feel lacking and inferior, what message do they send to those who are not defined as 'able-bodied'? If it is believed that everything can be fixed, that we can create 'perfection' and discard everything about us that is imperfect, what does this say about those who may be left behind in the genetic race to flawlessness?

Jeremy Rifkin says the development of new traits engineered into the foetus to improve certain capabilities – what he calls life-control technologies – gives tremendous extended power to the scientific establishment (Rifkin, 1998). And it won't just be attempts to change physical characteristics, modifying behaviour and thought are also in the sights of the bioengineers.

On the list of psychosomatic conditions and behavioural dispositions supposedly wholly or partly genetically determined, and therefore potentially genetically identifiable, are alcoholism, drug dependency, depression, shyness, aggressiveness, domestic violence, criminality and kleptomania. Our genes, so we are being told, give us a predisposition to Alzheimer's disease, diabetes, schizophrenia, asthma, homosexuality, ugliness and misanthropy. A 1996 study found a genetic basis for 'novelty seeking', 'thrill seeking', and 'excitability' along with 'restless impulsivity' and 'instant gratification' which, according to the study's authors, were factors in determining educational failure and criminality (Fisher, 1996).[58]

David Koshland, editor of *Science* magazine, even attributes homelessness and unemployment to genetic defects. He has suggested that common genetic diseases are at the root of many societal problems, the cost of which 'cries out for an early solution that involves prevention, not caretaking' (Koshland, 1989, p. 189). Again we hear echoes of a eugenic past when a person could be diagnosed with the genetic defect of being 'shiftless' and 'unattached'.[59]

The view that our fate is determined by our genes – genetic fatalism – leads to the logical conclusion that genetic intervention is inevitable. Why bother changing social conditions, why try to improve our environments, if it's really just a matter of altering and adjusting genes to get the kind of people we want populating the planet? Buchanan et al., in *From chance to choice: Genetics and justice*, observe:

> Individuals are not responsible for their behaviour (tiny chemical factories embedded within them are), nor are we responsible for critically evaluating and perhaps reforming existing institutions and social practices, since these are largely irrelevant to the problems that most concern us. If there were an all-powerful and all-knowing

being who was resolutely committed to shielding the existing social and political order from critical scrutiny, it is unlikely that it could hit upon a better strategy than implanting genetic determinist thinking in people's heads (2000, p. 24).

Francis Fukuyama, in *Our posthuman future*, warns that genetic determinist beliefs leading to genetic enhancement practices have dire repercussions for society:

> If wealthy parents suddenly have open to them the opportunity to increase the intelligence of their children as well as that of all their subsequent descendants, then we have the makings not just of a moral dilemma but of a full-scale class war (2002, p. 16).

Genes, destiny and discrimination

We see the fetishism of genes in popular culture.[60] Rothman has pointed out that genetics is no longer just a science or a set of technologies, but 'an ideology . . . the way we are more and more thinking about life . . .' (Rothman, 1998, p. 283). She says geneticists, in their descriptions of DNA, 'sound religious, awestruck, overwhelmed by the power and majesty of the DNA: It's the Bible, the Holy Grail, the Book of Man. Those are their very words' (Rothman, 1998, p. 284). They seem to be suffering delusions of biotech grandeur (Buchanan et al., 2000, p. 23). But the assumptions behind geneism are being questioned. Pioneers in the field of ecogenetics are finding gene after gene only acting as a 'bad seed' in the presence of some environmental factor.[61]

'What is a good gene and what is a bad gene depends on how you treat it,' said geneticist Charles Sing of the University of Michigan. 'Genes don't wake up until they are exposed to some environmental factor.' Sing counts himself 'among the growing number of conscientious objectors to the genes-as-destiny dogma' (in Begley, 1993, pp. 64–65). Richard Strohman of the

University of California, Berkeley, shares Sing's view: 'The presence of a genetic marker . . . is no guarantee that abnormality or disease will show up.'

> In many people *with* [italics in original] disease, moreover, tracing the malady to a gene is impossible: as many as 20 genes may be related to hypertension, at least three to manic depression and more than 100 to cancer.
>
> But the best news has nothing to do with brave new cures. It is, quite simply, that our future is not written indelibly in our genes. (in Begley, 1993, pp. 64–65).

The obsession with genes has caused many to forget the role of environment in triggering genetic problems. Joshua Lederberg, who received a Nobel Prize for his work in bacterial genetics, has estimated that environmental factors such as drugs, food additives and unclean air could account for eighty percent of the prevailing human mutation rate (Kevles, 1985, p. 288). As Rifkin observes:

> While each individual has varying genetic susceptibilities to these diseases, environmental factors, including diet and lifestyle, are major contributing elements that can trigger genetic mutations. Heavy cigarette smoking, high levels of alcohol consumption, diets rich in animal fats, the use of pesticides and other poisonous chemicals, contaminated water and food, polluted air, and sedentary living habits have been shown, in study after study, to cause genetic mutations and lead to the onset of many of these high-profile diseases (1998, pp. 228–229).

Genetic identity is beginning to establish itself as a defining category in the same way individuals are identified by their ethnic origins. As Edwin Black comments: 'Like eugenics, newgenics would begin by establishing genetic identity, which is already becoming a factor in society, much like ethnic identity and credit identity. DNA identity databanks are rapidly proliferating' (2003, p. 429).

As a result of assessing people according to their genetic makeup, they start being discriminated against on that basis. In a 1996 US study of 917 individuals, 455 reported that they had experienced some form of discrimination based on their genetic makeup and genetic predispositions, mostly by insurance companies and health providers. Examples include:

- A health maintenance organisation refused to pay for occupational therapy after an individual was diagnosed with MPS-I, arguing that it was a pre-existing condition.
- A 24-year-old woman was refused life insurance because her family had a history of Huntington's disease, despite the fact that she had never been tested for the disease.
- One family had its entire coverage cancelled when the insurance company discovered that one of its four children was afflicted with fragile X disease. The rest of the children were free of the disease but lost their coverage anyway.
- A couple was denied adoption because the wife was 'at risk' of coming down with Huntington's disease.
- A birth mother with Huntington's disease was not allowed to put up her child for adoption through a state adoption agency.
- Another couple, one of whom was at risk of developing Huntington's, was denied adoption of a normal baby but was allowed to adopt a baby at risk of coming down with Huntington's disease.

These examples point to the development of an 'informal genetic caste system', says Jeremy Rifkin. As he points out:

> The very idea that genetically 'at risk' couples should only be paired with genetically 'at risk' babies, and vice versa, is still another early warning sign of what might potentially develop into a kind of informal genetic caste system in the coming century (Rifkin, 1998, pp. 161, 163).[62]

'How dare you?': The defiance of disabled women

The ingrained view that life with a disability is not worth living is challenged by women in this book who have a disability and/or some type of disease or illness. Bearing in mind the ubiquitous assumption – whether open or hidden – that women with disabilities should not 'replicate their kind', their stories are particularly remarkable. And yet they don't want to be singled out as having done anything special – they've just chosen to take part in the joys and challenges of parenting like other people do, decided to get on with it and make the most of life.

But society's assumptions about them are difficult to shake. As E. Boylan writes in *Women and disability* (1991, p. 52), 'Disabled women are systematically denied the most human of rights – the right to love . . . marriage . . . motherhood' (in Kallianes & Rubenfeld, 1997, p. 211). Diane Coleman, President of Not Dead Yet, thinks it is because the very existence of disabled people is seen as a sign of societal failure. 'Medical professionals often have countless incorrect assumptions about our lives. Maybe they see us as failures on their part' (in Hershey, 1994, p. 29). Recalls Leisa Whitaker in her contribution in this book:

> . . . the specialist offered us an abortion. He asked us to think about whether we wanted to bring another dwarf baby into the world. It was something I hadn't even thought of. This was our baby! Why would we not want her? Why would the world not accept our child?

In a paper delivered to the Fourth Australian Women's Health Conference in 2001, disability activists Keren Howe and Carolyn Frohmader of Women With Disabilities Australia highlight a contradictory standard applied to women with disabilities:

> What is expected, encouraged and at times, compelled among non-disabled women is discouraged and proscribed for women with

disabilities. (As Leisa Whitaker says in her piece in this book you are made to feel you have to 'live by different rules.') Many women lose custody of their children in divorce, while others may have their children removed from their care by social welfare agencies, solely on the grounds that they have a disability (Howe & Frohmader, 2001, p. 203).

Howe and Frohmader cite a 1995 Australian study (Westbrook & Chinnery) which compared the child rearing experience of mothers with and without physical disabilities. The study found that:

- 36 percent of disabled women received negative reactions to their pregnancy from others, compared to 9 percent of the non-disabled women;
- 12 percent of the disabled women rated their doctors' care during pregnancy as 'poor' compared to 2 percent of the non-disabled women;
- 20 percent of the disabled women were advised by their doctor to have an abortion, compared to none of the non-disabled women;
- 23 percent of the disabled women found prenatal classes 'unhelpful' compared to 3 percent of the non-disabled women (reasons given by the disabled women as to why the classes were unhelpful included: lack of information; no consideration given to the needs of women with disabilities; feeling excluded in the classes);
- 24 percent of the disabled women found the maternity hospital staff 'unhelpful' compared to 7 percent of the non-disabled women (reasons given by the disabled women included: special needs of women with disabilities were ignored; patronising and bullying behaviour; rude and uncaring attitudes).

The reality of disabled women's lives has been compared to that of women from racial and ethnic minority groups, who are also disempowered and 'become scapegoats in a society that rations health care and other services' (Simpson, 1992, p. 8, cited in Kallianes & Rubenfeld, 1997, p. 211).

Victorian disability activist Kathleen Ball, in *Don't deliver us from disability*, states: 'Women with disabilities continue to be sterilised and when we do reproduce, over one third of our children are removed from our care' (in Newell, 2002, p. 16). Melissa Madsen (1993, p. 15) concurs: 'We have historically been on the receiving end of eugenicist sterilisation campaigns, and indeed sterilisation of girls and women with disability continues.'[63]

Anne Finger tells of disabled women who were asked, 'How did you get pregnant?' as though they could not possibly be capable of human love, as though having a disability rendered their reproductive systems dysfunctional (1984, p. 291, in Kallianes & Rubenfeld 1997, p. 206). Such a question also assumes they could not possibly parent children, a notion well dismissed in anthologies like *Bigger than the sky: Disabled women on parenting* (Wates & Jade, 1999).

Deborah Kaplan says in 'Disability rights: Perspectives on reproductive technologies and public policy', that physicians often counsel disabled women not to have children merely because it seemed obvious that people with disabilities would not make good parents (1998, p. 242). Donna Hyler writes that her gynaecologist and parents suggested she should not continue her pregnancy because the child would 'suffer psychological damage as a result of having a disabled parent' (1985, p. 282, in Kallianes & Rubenfeld, 1997, p. 209). The Family Planning worker in Jo Litwinowicz's story in this book is another example of this attitude:

> She calmly went on, 'You do realise that when your child can walk and talk it will come to you and say, "I hate you mother because you can't talk properly, you dribble and you're in a wheelchair and I want a new mother."'

B. Waxman contends that the disabled woman who becomes pregnant is judged to be immoral and society seeks to punish her by removing her child(ren) from her: 'While a nondisabled woman's pregnancy is considered a miracle, a disabled woman's pregnancy is considered a crime against society' (Waxman, 1993, p. 6). Indeed, Julie Park and Belinda Strookappe document this discriminatory attitude in their study of New Zealand haemophiliacs. 'You should not have children, how dare you!' was the response of a health professional to a couple who refused coercive counselling (Park & Strookappe, 1996, p. 64).

Is it wrong for women with disabilities and illnesses (such as haemophilia and HIV) to find in this echoes of Justice Holmes's injunction that 'society can prevent those who are manifestly unfit from continuing their kind'? Is it wrong for them to feel slighted every time disability is used to justify abortion, even up to birth; for 'foetal abnormality' to be the virtually unquestioned category which extends any limits on abortion? (It is instructive to note how amniocentesis has been used to extend the upper limits of pregnancy at which abortion can lawfully take place.)[64]

How do people with disabilities feel when those like L. M. Purdy, in an article titled 'Genetic diseases: Can having children be immoral?', write of the necessity of 'preventing the existence of miserable beings . . . To see the genetic line continued entails a sinister legacy of illness and death' (Purdy, 1978, p. 314). Disability activist Adriene Asch tells us how it feels:

> . . . prenatal diagnosis and selective termination communicate that disability is so terrible that it warrants not being alive . . . As a society, do we wish to send the message to all such people now living that there should be no more of your kind in the future?' (Asch, 1989, p. 319).

Leisa Whitaker and her family got sent that message when a

32-week-old unborn baby girl with suspected dwarfism was aborted at Royal Women's Hospital in Melbourne, Australia. She, her husband, and four children have this condition. So does Frances Allen who wrote to *The Age*:

> . . . I have Turner's syndrome, which causes short stature. I am not as short as people [with] dwarfism but I am shorter than my school friends. I am 17 but about the height of a 13-year-old. I can't believe that someone who can lead a normal, happy, healthy life could be aborted because of how they look. When I was diagnosed with Turner's syndrome a few years ago, I was given a book to read. I was absolutely shocked to read that a great number of pregnancies were aborted if found to have Turner's syndrome. As I was 14 when I found out, I know I am completely normal – apart from the fact that I am extremely short. I was shocked to think that I might have been aborted. The baby that was aborted could have lead [*sic*] a normal happy life, and if the parents didn't want it there would have been plenty of people willing to adopt it and bring it up as theirs. Foetuses should not be aborted due to their appearance. This baby did not have a life threatening disease or problem – its only problem was its short stature. Once born it could have led a happy, healthy life . . . (Allen, 2000, p. 9).

Ravi Savarirayan, a clinical geneticist, told *The Age* he had more than twenty calls from short-statured people, many saying they were afraid or ashamed to go outside because 'they felt society didn't want them to be around.' As one patient walked down the street, a man yelled from a car: 'You should have been aborted' (in Toy & Milburn, 2000, p. 3).

What is normal?

Who is to judge what is normal? As more and more conditions and so-called imperfections become detectable, as the range of what is considered unacceptable broadens, as new eugenic ideas such as those we've seen above take root, more babies will be selected out. Already, abortions have been carried out for correctible conditions. For example, in Australia, abortion provider Dr David Grundmann has admitted performing abortions after twenty weeks gestation for cleft lip and palate.[65] Already it has become acceptable to use preimplantation diagnosis to screen out embryos of the wrong sex for 'family balancing' purposes.[66]

As Maguire and McGee put it, today's normal might be seen as subnormal, leading to the medicalisation of another area of life (Maguire & McGee, 1999).

When a hearing parent said, 'I have a right to want surgery for my child which will make him more like me, a hearing person,' Gary Malkowski, then legislator in Ontario, Canada, replied, 'Then presumably you have no objection to deaf parents requesting surgery to make their child deaf' (in Campbell, 2000, p. 309).

So, here they are, 19 women from different parts of the world, who have said no to conformity and yes to diversity; who have refused to allow themselves and their babies to be excised from the mainland of humanity, who confronted impersonal technologies of quality control with strength and dignity.

Notes

Introduction

1. A 'disability phobic' society, in the words of Kallianes and Rubenfeld (1997). Disabled Women and Reproductive Rights.
2. This phrase is used in Spallone, P. (1992). *Generation games: Genetic engineering and the future for our lives*. It is attributed to Nancy Wexler, 'Will the circle be unbroken?' (1980).
3. I have borrowed the term 'bad babies' from Finger, A. (1984). Claiming all of our bodies: reproductive rights and disabilities.

4. Lippman, A. (1991). Prenatal genetic testing and screening: constructing needs and reinforcing inequities. Lippman cites Rothman, B.K. (1989). *Recreating motherhood: Ideology and technology in a patriarchal society*, who quotes a doctor in the childbirth movement as using the description 'blue ribbon baby'.
5. Less than 15 percent of disorders detected through prenatal tests can be treated. Rifkin, J. (1998). *The biotech century*.
6. Note how the headlines trumpet 'cures' for all kinds of conditions without mentioning that the so-called cure is not eliminating a disease, but eliminating the bearer of a disease. Richard Lewontin states this clearly: 'To conflate . . . the prevention of *disease* with the prevention of *lives* that will involve disease, is to traduce completely the meaning of preventive medicine . . . Genetic counselling and selective abortion are substitutes for disease prevention and cure.' Lewontin, R. C. (1997, March 6). Science & 'the demon-haunted world': An exchange cited in Buchanan et al. (2000) *From chance to choice: Genetics and justice* [italics in original].

The medical gaze

7. Cara Dunne and Catherine Warren argue 'wrongful termination suits' should be brought to challenge the 'unfounded nature of . . . wrongful birth cases'.

   This . . . would be brought on behalf of aggrieved parents who were compelled by the advice and information of their medical providers to terminate their pregnancy. Their injury was the loss of an individual whom they later learned would have had a manageable condition . . . In justifiably relying on the information provided, they allege their reproductive right to bear a child with a disability was violated and they seek pain and suffering damages (1998, pp. 197, 199).

8. See also Lupton, D. (1999). Risk and the ontology of pregnant embodiment, and Scioscia, A. (1999). Prenatal genetic diagnosis.

Genetic screening in context: Towards a eugenics civilization

9. 'Eugenically superior' eggs were sold for up to $50,000 in an internet auction in 1999. Arent, L. (1999). Serving up eggs on the web.
10. See, for example, Tuch et al. (2003). Use of human fetal tissue for biomedical research in Australia 1994–2002.
11. I've borrowed 'biological pluralism and the elimination of genetic variations' from Justice Michael Kirby's introduction in Goggin, G. & Newell, C. (2005). *Disability in Australia: Exposing a social apartheid*.
12. A 1994 study of 161,560 foetuses showed 86 percent of women who found out they were carrying a baby with Down syndrome elected to abort, according to Harvard Medical School professor Lewis B. Holmes, senior

author of the study conducted by researchers from Massachusetts General Hospital and Brigham and Women's Hospital.

13. Kass elaborates on much of this more recently in Kass, L. R. (2002). *Life, liberty and the defense of dignity: The challenge for bioethics.*

Lack of choice and the coercive power of testing

14. The authors of a 1995 UK study support this view:

> Women who decline the offer of testing are seen as having more control over this outcome, and are attributed more blame for it, than are women who have not been offered tests and also give birth to a child with Down syndrome . . . The results of the current study would suggest that less help will be given to parents who decline testing because the outcome, giving birth to a child with a condition for which prenatal screening and selective termination are available, is seen as preventable.
>
> Marteau, T. M. & Drake, H. (1995, p. 1130). Attributions for disability: The influence of genetic screening.

The routinisation of testing

15. Santalahti et al. (1998), in On what grounds do women participate in prenatal screening? state that respect for women's autonomy and informed decision making requires that women should be told that ultrasound screening can lead to them having to make a decision about abortion (p. 162).

16. Beech, B. & Anderson, G. (1999). We went through psychological hell: A case report of prenatal diagnosis. When the couple realised what was actually going to happen, they refused to terminate.

17. Natalie Withers' story was part of a Channel Nine (Australia) *60 Minutes* program on late-term abortion, 'The Great Debate', on 17 April 2005.

The right to choose not to know

18. Clarkeburn also describes selective abortion as a 'preventative' method.

19. Kolker and Burke (1994) have a different view of knowledge, especially when information is unexpected:

> Knowledge does not always empower; instead, it may confuse and paralyse. Parents may have to contend with perhaps the most unforseen consequence of all: too much information, that is information they never realized the testing might yield and information they are not emotionally equipped to handle (p. 165).

20. After being made to feel alarmed (including by a receptionist) about the results, a second opinion at another medical facility found the predictions for her child unfounded, and her son was later born healthy. Beech, B. & Anderson, G. (1999). We went through psychological hell: A case report of prenatal diagnosis.

The 'benevolent tyranny of expertise'

21. Green, J. M. (1993). Ethics and late termination of pregnancy. Green concludes: 'Clarification of the law is needed so that obstetricians realise that they can terminate beyond 24 weeks for conditions that they judge to be serious' (p. 1179). The 1993 survey of 391 obstetric consultants in the UK sought their views on how late they would be prepared to offer termination of pregnancy for anencephaly, spina bifida and Down syndrome. A total of 89 percent of consultants said they would offer termination for anencephaly at 24 weeks, 60 percent would offer termination for Down syndrome at 24 weeks and 13 percent after 24 weeks. For open spina bifida, 21 percent would provide abortion after 24 weeks. A total of 75 percent of clinical geneticists and obstetricians specialising in ultrasound believed termination should be available for dwarfism at 24 weeks.

22. See Tankard Reist, M. (2004a). No amount of hand wringing will bring back dead babies after abortion.

23. See, for example, Gevers, S. (1999). Third trimester abortion for fetal abnormality.

24. From collected email correspondence in journal of Teresa Streckfuss, 30 May 2001.

No assessment of the cost to women's health

25. See Hunfeld et al. (1995). The grief of late pregnancy loss; Hunfeld, J. A. et al. (1994). Pregnancy termination, perceived control, and perinatal grief; Lloyd, J. & Laurence, K. M. (1985). Sequelae and support after termination of pregnancy for fetal malformation, and Furlong, R. & Black, R. (1984). Pregnancy termination for genetic indications: The impact on families. See also Leithner et al. (2004). Affective state of women following a prenatal diagnosis: predictors of a negative psychological outcome. They comment:

> The active decision to terminate a wanted pregnancy following an adverse prenatal diagnosis as well as any loss of a pregnancy . . . frequently result in acute feelings of grief, despair and guilt, and may also cause severe long-term psychological sequelae (p. 240).

> Leithner et al. also observe: '[W]omen facing a prenatal diagnosis experience considerable psychological distress, which may be underestimated by workers in prenatal care' (2004, p. 244).

Questions about risks of ultrasound and amniocentesis

26. See Brookes, A. (1994). Women's experience of routine prenatal ultrasound. pp. 1–5.

Agonising decisions based on questionable findings

27. This is the same doctor who has defended the abortion of a 32-week unborn baby with suspected dwarfism (see Tankard Reist, M., 2004a).

Lack of knowledge among medical professionals

28. The authors provide a disturbing example of this variation in understanding and information provided to parents:

> One health professional considered 47XXX to be 'as devastating as Down syndrome' and said 'that there was a possibility of mental retardation, intelligence down, stunted.' Another health professional who considered 47XXX to be a very mild condition told parents that: 'She would be a perfectly normal baby and she would go to a school, a normal school, and she would grow up normally and that she had an extra chromosome . . . [I] explained to them that the child would look just like every other child and that she was a normal child and that her intelligence might not be quite as great as you would expect for her parents but that she would still cope in a normal school.
>
> Abramsky et al. (2001, p. 465). What parents are told after prenatal diagnosis of a sex chromosome abnormality.

'They turn the baby into a monster!': Lack of information on disability and support

29. Dunne, C. & Warren, C. (1998). Lethal autonomy: The malfunction of the informed consent mechanism within the context of prenatal diagnosis of genetic variants. Dunne and Warren describe an 'imbalance in information provision which is skewing patient decision toward eugenic targeting of disabled children . . .' (p. 201). They want it redressed through mandatory education of genetic professionals in law, education policy and resource networks as they relate to disability and propose genetic counsellors be required to undertake internships with foundations, school programs and community service organisations. A strong example of the lack of non-directiveness within the medical profession is given in Whiteside, R. K. & Perry, D. L. (2001). Stereotype, segregate and eliminate: 'Disability', selective abortion and the context of 'choice'. National Council on Intellectual Disability. Foetal medicine specialist Janet Vaughan relates that when she phoned doctors with the results of their patients' tests, they often say, 'Oh, well, have you told her what to do?' Vaughan responds that that's not her job. They respond, 'Oh, so I've got to do it, have I?' (p. 24).

30. Blumberg, L. (1994b). The politics of prenatal testing and selective abortion. Blumberg quotes Finnegan, J. (1991). Relinquishing a child for special needs adoption: Prenatal diagnosis and pregnancy options. Blumberg observes: 'Even if it is assumed that the parents who are most likely to inquire about adoption are those with a bias against pregnancy termination, these figures should give traditional genetic counsellors reason to pause' (p. 145).

31. Baby Doe and Baby Jane Doe are two of the most well-known cases involving the withdrawal of treatment and nutrition from babies with disabilities (who were not terminally ill). Infant Doe was allowed to starve to death over six days because she had Down syndrome. Baby Jane Doe was born with spina bifida but denied treatment because doctors predicted severe physical handicap and mental retardation if she was allowed to live. However she did not die and functions normally, though not as well as she would have, had surgery not been denied her (Dunne, C. & Warren, C. 1998, p. 174). Lethal autonomy: The malfunction of the informed consent mechanism within the context of prenatal diagnosis of genetic variants.

Dehumanising and stigmatising labels

32. Her son, Jonti, was born without the condition.
33. There are a number of reported cases of babies being born alive after termination. Helen Parker was told to abort at 22 weeks due to severe pre-eclampsia. The baby survived the abortion and is now one year old (Laing, L., 2004). The baby who would not let go. See also Jansen, R. P. S. (1990). Unfinished feticide.
34. Zamichow, N. (1995). Newsletter articles stir furore in high-IQ group, and Cooper, A. (1995). Remember what the social engineers wrought. Similar attitudes are displayed towards those of certain races. Tony Bouza, a Minneapolis *Star Tribune* columnist, claimed in 1989 that abortion was needed for the 'at risk' population: 'poor, black and Indian' whose children are 'marked for failure' (Bouza, T., 1989). A mother's day wish: Make abortion available to all women. Even more recently, a contributor to a white supremacist site wrote of her misgivings about abortion – except when the babies were coloured:

> Ever since I became racially aware I've been of two minds regarding abortion. On the one hand I find it to be reprehensible (especially partial-birth abortion). But on the other hand I am loyal to my race and if I follow my racial loyalty to its logical conclusion the position I end up with concerning abortion is that the legality of abortion should depend on the race of the child. No white child should ever be aborted. The planet is crawling with blacks, browns and yellows . . . we don't need any more of them. Abortion of these children should be legal if not encouraged outright. (Stormfront White Nationalist Community: www.stormfront.org)

The rise of eugenicist thought

35. There are a number of thorough and fascinating works on the history of eugenics. I mention only a few here, on which I drew for this section: Kevles, D. J. (1985). *In the name of eugenics: Genetics and the uses of human heredity*, is a detailed account of eugenics from Galton onwards; Thom, D.

& Jennings, M. (1996), Human pedigree and the 'best stock': From eugenics to genetics? provide a useful history of the origins of eugenics primarily in the UK; Galton, D. (2001), *In our own image: Eugenics and the genetic modification of people*; Rosen, C. (2004), *Preaching eugenics: Religious leaders and the American eugenics movement.*

    Some papers on eugenic thought in Australia (including papers documenting efforts to 'breed out the colour' of the Indigenous population, and surf culture and eugenics – They ride the surf like gods: Sydney-side beach culture, life-saving and eugenics, 1902–1940) – can be found in Crotty et al., *A race for a place* (2000). See also Buchanan et al., *From chance to choice: Genetics and justice* (2000) (though I do not agree with the broader position of their book, especially with their view about the legitimate role of the state in pursuing eugenic policies in the future).

36. See Laughlin, H. (1914) [superintendent, Eugenics Record Office, Cold Springs Harbor, Long Island, New York], Calculations on the working out of a proposed program of sterilization, in *Proceedings of the First National Conference on Race Betterment*, January 8–12, 1914.

37. A compelling account of the history of coercive sterilisation is found in Trombley, S. (1988). *The right to reproduce: A history of coercive sterilization.* This book was removed from bookshelves as a result of legal threats from Planned Parenthood.

38. Years after Carrie gave birth to Vivian, she claimed the father was a nephew of the Dobbses, who had raped her (see Black, 2003, p. 109).

39. Sadly, Carrie's sister, Doris Buck Figgins, was also sterilised at Lynchburg, in 1928 – tricked into it by being told she needed to have her appendix removed. When Doris learned the truth, 'I broke down and cried. My husband and me wanted children desperate – were crazy about them. I never knew what they'd done to me' (in Trombley, S., 1988, p. 91). *The right to reproduce: A history of coercive sterilization.*

40. Missing letters and words in original typescript. It is unclear why she is referred to as 'Mrs W'.

41. Comments Trombley (p. 243): 'Apart from the general horror of the tone of the board, two points are worthy of note. Firstly, Mrs W. was neither feeble-minded nor epileptic, so the assumption that her child might be either was totally unfounded; and secondly, the questioner's tone is quite menacing when he says to Mrs W., 'if you live, you may want to marry and set up a home'.

42. A British social worker, Moya Woodside, wrote *Sterilization in North Carolina; A sociological and psychological study* (1950), one of the key texts in the promotion of eugenic sterilisation. In it, she considers why the less educated 'are slow to accept new ideas, and incapable of viewing a situation except in immediate personal terms'. Trombley writes:

Woodside observes that of the eighty-five county welfare departments she questioned, seventy-one of them noted that resistance of clients and relatives was 'a major problem'. In her post-sterilization survey, Woodside encountered women who regretted the operation. Her method of dealing with this was to diagnose the women as maladjusted: '. . . where unfavourable results were observed, they were associated with neurotic personality and maladjustment in the life situation.'

See Trombley, S. (1988, p. 170). *The right to reproduce: A history of coercive sterilization*. Attempts are being made in North Carolina, USA, to provide cash reparations to victims of eugenic sterilisation. State legislator Rep. Larry Womble has filed legislation asking the state to make payments to surviving victims of the North Carolina eugenics program which was active from 1929 to 1974. An estimated 7600 people were sterilised under the program which was the third largest in the US after California and Virginia (Begos & Ingram, 2005, April 24). The Bill would offer cash reparations to victims of eugenic sterilisation.

Birth control and eugenics

43. For an account of how pre-war eugenicists influenced the development of public health and family planning in Australia, see Wyndham, D. (1997). *Striving for national fitness: Eugenics in Australia 1910s to 1930s*.

44. Black, E. (2003). *War against the weak*. See Black for details of Sanger's work outlining this position.

45. Class and race prejudices came unsubtly to the fore in the labels used by mainstream eugenicists. In 1921, Marie Stopes spoke of 'that intolerable stream of misery which ever overflows its banks'; others chose descriptions like 'social pests', 'sewerage', 'scum' and 'waste humanity', and warned that society was 'breeding degenerate hordes of a demoralized "residuum" unfit for social life' (in Buchanan et al., 2000. *From chance to choice: Genetics and justice* p. 44). In 1936 Madison Grant, author of *The passing of the great race*, labelled what he saw as the insuperior masses, 'human flotsam', quoted in Black, E. (2003). *War against the weak*.

46. It has never ceased to puzzle me that an international abortion provider chose the name of Marie Stopes, an unrepentant eugenicist, as the banner for its enterprise.

Eugenics and extermination

47. United States Holocaust Memorial Museum, Washington DC (http://www.holocaust-trc.org/hndcp.htm). Operation T4 was the code name reference for Tiergartenstrasse 4, the address of the Berlin Chancery Offices, where the program was headquartered. See United States Holocaust Memorial Museum, http://www.holocaust-trc.org/hndcp.htm.

The new 'nice' eugenics

48. Rakowski, E. (2002). Who should pay for bad genes?:

> The government could reward people who availed themselves of those services in exactly the same way as the private organisation, Project Prevention, pays cash to former drug addicts or alcoholics who undergo permanent sterilization or who use certain long-term contraceptives. The government might require couples to undergo tests before marriage, it could go one step further and mandate mutual disclosure of the results. Or the government might, through legal permission or financial subsidy, make post-conception interventions possible, such as in utero corrective therapy or abortion. Finally, the government might penalize intentional or reckless conduct either directly, by fining parents or imposing criminal sanctions, or indirectly, by empowering children to sue for wrongful life (p. 1408).

For an account of the current practice of enticing drug-addicted women to undergo sterilisation in the US, see Hodgson, M. (2005, May 14). Glynis Anderson, now director of a recovery centre near Detroit, describes how her children were her motivation to get off drugs:

> I am a recovering addict, and if it was not for my children, I wouldn't be clean today. They were my motivation to get better ... It's easy to blame the addict, but people can get clean, and a large percentage do it for their children. It'd be a hell of a thing to regret, wouldn't it? Not being able to have children, for 200 bucks (in Hodgson, 2005, p. 42).

Testing and termination as a bargain: 'Units of handicapped prevented'

49. Harris et al. continue (pp. 280–281):

> In addition to providing information about fetal chromosomal status to the pregnant woman, prenatal testing avoids subsequent costs associated with raising a child affected by Down's syndrome or another trisomy ... We used an additional incremental lifetime cost of $228,400 per child with a trisomy, calculated by weight averaging the cost of each trisomy by its prevalence.
>
> ... our findings suggest that prenatal diagnosis should be offered to pregnant women irrespective of age or risk (because such testing can be cost effective, depending on the woman's preferences), and that special attention should be paid to the preferences of the individual on offering such testing, including the desired level of reassurance the patient needs (because individual preferences can greatly affect the cost utility of testing).

Note how 'the women's preferences' suddenly get a mention in the article, perhaps to take the edge off the economic rationalist approach with its 'incremental lifetime cost' assessment per child.

50. Cara Dunne and Catherine Warren relate an intervention at the 46th Annual Conference of the American Society of Human Genetics, at which the Professional Practice and Guidelines Committee of the American Medical College of Genetics sought criteria to measure what would constitute a 'successful outcome' in the national Tay Sachs genetic counselling

and screening program, for the purposes of a grant. A scientist protested: 'We can't just measure success in terms of detected defective fetuses which have been aborted?' To which the Director of the Tay Sachs screening program at the University of California at San Diego, Michael Kaybeck, who presided over the committee, responded, 'Why can't we? . . . We cannot think of our program as eliminating defective children. We must think of it as allowing for the births of many, many healthy, unaffected children' (in Dunne, C. & Warren, C., 1998, pp. 171–172). Lethal autonomy: The malfunction of the informed consent mechanism within the context of prenatal diagnosis of genetic variants.

The quest for perfection and the gospel of gene salvation

51. See Brooks, L. (1998). All for the breast; Burkham, C. (2005). Nip and tuck nation pp. 24–26; Armitage, C. (2003). Stretching their legs, pp. 30–33.
52. See also Savulescu, J. (2005). It's our duty to make better babies. p. 19, and Dunne, A. & Noble, T. (2005). Should science reshape the human race?
53. A number of experiments mixing human and animal DNA have taken place already. One was conducted in Australia in 2000 when the Australian biotech company Stem Cell Sciences and the American company Biotransplant made a pig–human embryo by inserting a human somatic foetal cell into the egg of a pig, which was developed, according to the patent application, to the 32-cell stage. Peter Mountford of Stem Cell Sciences claimed the embryos could have been implanted in a woman or a sow. See Smith, W. J. (2004). *Consumer's Guide to a brave new world*, Benson, S. (2001b). Australia: Human clone trials – Secret DNA cell testing revealed, p. 9, and Benson, S. (2001a). Australia: Dark side when life imitates life. p. 19. In 2003 a US-trained scientist in China revealed she had fused human chromosomes with rabbit eggs, creating 400 cross-species embryos, developing 100 to the blastocyst stage, and a US fertility expert created between 600 and 700 cow–human hybrids, developing 200 to the blastocyst stage (Cook, M. 2003). Human experiments threaten dignity, p. 18. In June 2005, Australian Professor Alan Trounson called for cloning laws to be relaxed to allow scientists to create diseased human embryos from which to extract stem cells for research. Noble, T. (2005, June 5). Let us create diseased stem cells – Researcher. pp. 1–2.

Such experiments make one wonder if there are any limits. In July 2003, US scientists created hybrid human 'she-males', mixing male and female cells in the same embryo and claiming the research could lead to cures for genetic disorders. See Henderson, M. (2003). Scientists create mixed-sex embryos, and Reuters (2003). Creation of human 'she-males' sparks outrage.
54. Pence, G. (1998). *Who's afraid of human cloning?* cited in Smith, W. J. (2004), *Consumer's Guide to a brave new world*. Smith explains how cloning could be

used to genetically enhance a child. Cells will be extracted from a donor and the DNA in the nucleus genetically engineered to taste, and then used in human SCNT cloning. Once the cloned embryo reaches the blastocyst stage – five to seven days of development – it is implanted into a woman's womb and gestated to birth. The child's genes will be virtually identical in genetic makeup to the modified cell from which s/he received almost their entire DNA. In theory, this would result in the child exhibiting the desired 'enhancements'.

Another supporter of this process is Martin Lishexian Lee, who writes that cloning has 'a genetic health effect by enabling the choice of better genes to copy or modify' (Lee, 2004). The Inadequacies of Absolute Prohibition of Reproductive Cloning.

55. On April 28, 2005, the UK House of Lords approved of the Human Fertilisation & Embryology Authority granting a licence for the production of a child, who had been screened so as to be able to provide 'clean stem cells' for the treatment of a sick older brother, now six.

56. 'Killing a disabled infant is not morally equivalent to killing a person. Very often it is not wrong at all' (Singer, P. 1979). *Practical ethics*. See also Kuhse, H. & Singer, P. (1985). *Should the baby live?* and Singer, P. (1995). Killing babies isn't always wrong. pp. 20–22. A number of hospitals are putting the Singer philosophy into action. A *Lancet* report says that more than half of the newborn babies who died in Belgium between August 1999 and July 2000 died due to the withholding or withdrawing of treatment. In 40 cases out of 253, opiate pain killers were used in lethal doses (Australasian Bioethics Information, 2005, April 1); Belgian doctors often kill newborns (*BioEdge* Issue 154). An Associated Press article (December 2, 2004) reported that a hospital in the Netherlands has been administering lethal doses of sedatives to disabled newborns. *New York Sun* columnist Alicia Colon wrote of these killings: 'What the Groningen Academic Hospital is doing is fulfilling the nonvoluntary euthanasia that . . . Singer has been propounding for years.' (Colon, A., 2004, p. 2). When killing an infant is not wrong. See also Wesley J. Smith (2003). Continent Death: Euthanasia in Europe.

57. World Transhumanist Association. James Hughes declares: 'Let the ruling classes and Luddites tremble at a democratic transhumanist revolution. Would-be genemods and cyborgs! You have nothing to lose but your human bodies, and longer lives and bigger brains to win! TRANSHUMANISTS OF ALL COUNTRIES, UNITE!' [Capitals in original.] Hughes, J. (n.d.). *Democratic Transhumanism*.

58. See also Rifkin, J. (1998). *The biotech century*; Germov, J. (2000). 'My genes made me do it': A sociology of the 'new genetics'. Galton devotes a chapter

to the issue of genes and personality traits in Galton, D. (2001). *In our own image: Eugenics and the genetic modification of people.*

59. In Virginia in the 1920s, the conditions of feeblemindedness and epilepsy were considered synonymous with a condition diagnosed as shiftlessness: 'the genetic defect of being worthless and unattached in life'; Smith, J. D. & Nelson, K. R. (1989), quoted in Black, E. (2003). *War against the weak.*

Genes, destiny and discrimination

60. Buchanan et al. (2000). *From chance to choice: Genetics and justice* (p. 23) cite Lindee, S. & Nelkin, D. (1995) *The DNA mystique: The gene as a cultural icon*, as 'eloquently documenting' this.

61. For a scientific explanation of how genes work see Sober, E. (2000). Appendix One: The meaning of genetic causation. In A. Buchanan et al. (Eds.) (2000). *From chance to choice: Genetics and justice* (pp. 347–368).

62. For a broad examination of the issue, see Protection of human genetic information, Issues Paper 26, Australian Law Reform Commission and Australian Health Ethics Committee, Commonwealth of Australia, October 2001.

'How dare you?': The defiance of disabled women

63. See also Women with Disabilities Australia (WWDA) in Association with the Disability Studies and Research Institute (DSARI) and Lee Ann Basser (2004); Submission to the Commonwealth and state/territory governments regarding non-therapeutic sterilisation of minors with a decision-making disability, and Brady et al. (2001). *The sterilisation of girls and young women with a disability: Issues and progress.*

64. The availability of amniocentesis 'influenced legislation so that the upper limit of gestational age for legally tolerated termination of pregnancy was adjusted to the requirements of second trimester prenatal diagnosis in several countries' (Fuhrmann, W., 1989, pp. 378–385). Impact, logistics and prospects of traditional prenatal diagnosis.

What is normal?

65. Queensland Parliament Hansard (1995, October 31) "Grundmann Clinic – September: AMA Working Party"; Newsletter of the Queensland branch of the World Federation of Doctors who Respect Human Life, September 1995, p. 7. See also Tankard Reist, M. (2004c). Take a look at late-term abortions.

66. See Padawer, R. (2005, May 3). Sex selection of babies forces new debate. In this piece, David King, director of the UK Human Genetics Alert, describes sorting embryos on the basis of their sex as 'the exercise of sexism at the most profound level'.

The United Kingdom Parliament Select Committee on Science and Technology Fifth Report found, 'On balance we find no adequate justification for prohibiting the use of sex selection for family balancing.' Conclusions and Recommendations, no 30.

Sydney IVF in Australia has advertised its IVF services as available for 'family balancing' purposes. In 2002, it provided gender selection 'for purely social reasons' to 120 couples; six out of ten using PGD did so for non-medical reasons (see Taylor, Z., 2003, p. 6). The price of a baby girl: $14,000 for the chance to choose your child's sex (Teutsch, D. 2003, March 9, p. 30). Michelle or Michael? How you can pick sex of baby.

Berkowitz & Snyder comment on sex selection techniques:

> [Sex selection] forces parents to figure sex into the calculus of a child's worth, to place a value on sex. Furthermore, by making a choice, parents must essentially prefer one sex over another . . . sex selection represents sexism in its purest . . . form as prior to conception . . . before parents can possibly know anything about their child, a child's worth is based in large part upon their sex (1998, p. 33).

Some disability rights activists point to hypocrisy in condemning pre-implantation diagnosis on the basis of sex, while agreeing with using it to detect and eliminate embryos with certain conditions. Writes Wolbring:

> The argument used is that sex selection would be an inherently discriminatory use of preimplantation diagnostics. Indeed it would be but it would be in the same way an inherently discriminatory use of preimplantation diagnostics if we use it to select for certain abilities or deselect based on a lack of abilities. However it seems that discrimination is not equal discrimination. An 'animal farm' philosophy and atmosphere and a double morality seems to exist in the argument of many of the 'non-disabled' NGOs and others who defend the prohibition of sex selection but do not defend and demand at the same time the prohibition of 'disability deselection'. It seems as long as something is labeled as 'medical use' and as something, which targets diseases, disabilities, and defects the inherently discriminatory use of a technology is allowed.

> Wolbring, G. (2003) NBIC, NGO's society and three types of disabled people.

Campbell, F. (2000). Eugenics in a different key? New technologies and the 'conundrum' of 'disability'. Campbell cites Lane, H. (1992). *The mask of benevolence: Disabling the deaf community.*

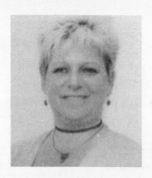

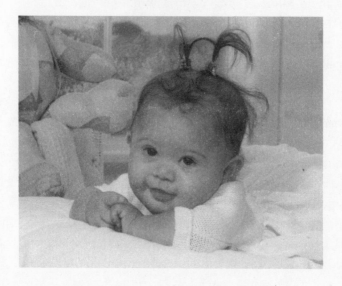

d.a.marullo

d.a.marullo has worked as a nurse and educator and counsellor for people with developmental delays for the past twenty-five years. She is a special needs advocate for children and adults. A mother of five children ranging in age from 28 to 2, she gained her Bachelor's Degree in English at the age of 40 and has completed teachers' college and high school creative writing and journalism courses. She lives in southern California where she is owned by her two cats.

d.a.marullo

THE STORY OF LAYIAH: MY WONDER CHILD

The party is over. Everyone has left and Layiah and her siblings are sound asleep. It was quite a rambunctious birthday party. Hard to believe she is 2 years old. It really went fast. I decided to sit down and write about the birth of my wonder child. So here's the whole story about how she almost didn't even come to be.

* * *

It was a warm breezy June night here in Southern California. We decided to go to dinner to celebrate our shared birthdays and the signing of our divorce papers that afternoon. I picked a quaint Italian restaurant in Santa Monica right on the pier. We had a sumptuous dinner of calamari and eggplant parmigiana and a complementary glass of chablis for dessert along with the New York cheesecake. We took a walk along the pier afterwards and decided to have one last fling together for old time's sake

Exactly one month later I went to the doctor for my regular diabetes checkup. My blood sugar was a little high, my blood pressure was good – and I was pregnant. What? The doctor was crazy. No way could I possibly be pregnant! I didn't even date yet! Then it dawned on me – the whole birthday dinner and the last fling with my ex. I quickly left the office and made another appointment with a different doctor. Same results. After the third doctor and a very frantic feeling deep inside, I had to give in to the fact that I was indeed pregnant from that one last fling.

I told no one. I expected to miscarry as I had in the past, anyway.

After eight weeks of still being pregnant, I saw a few specialists, all mandatory due to my age at the time: 44.

First there was the ultrasound that revealed that I was about seven to eight weeks pregnant. I even saw the little shadow on the film. It was bizarre. Deep inside I wanted it to be all a big mistake – you know – a tumor that they could remove and all would be well again. Then I was directed to the genetic counsellor, who basically sat me down and told me every possible terrible thing that could occur with this pregnancy, for 40 minutes straight. She advised terminating the pregnancy due to my 'point scale' (used to determine just how severe the problems could be with the pregnancy, taking into account age, family history and tests). She was advising termination of a life by a point scale! I wondered where I stood on that point scale, having so many things wrong with me and all; maybe it would be advisable to terminate me!

I then went back to have another ultrasound, this time by an expert in the field of difficult pregnancies. I wondered how they could label my pregnancy 'difficult' when nothing conclusive was proven yet! Anyway, I shuffled into this office only to find a young Latina girl crying and sobbing into a tissue. I asked her, in my terrible Spanish/English if there was anything that I could do, when she looked up and told me the doctor had advised she end her pregnancy due to the ultrasound that suggested her baby had a tubal defect. I wanted to tell her that that is not positive proof and that she needs way more tests, but I was already called into the examining room. As I lay there in the dark, technician and doctor attentively watching the screen before them, I wondered about that young girl and why anyone would suggest termination without having much of anything but an ultrasound to go by.

I was told to get dressed; I left that room to be ushered into a smaller room. The doctor came in and very matter-of-factly told me that my age and the possibility of defects were large enough warning signs that I should terminate. I objected to his reasoning and said that he was too quick to make such a vital decision.

He asked if I was having an amniocentesis test and I answered no. He said I should and then they could be sure of what he was sure of already and then I could terminate. I was appalled by this cold, horrible man standing before me. Did he not realise he was discussing a life inside me?

When I told him I had no intention of aborting, terminating or ending this pregnancy, I was surprised at my own voice and my strong conviction. He said that I would be sorry about the decision and that I only had a few weeks left to rethink it. I left so quickly that I forgot the book I'd brought to read. I cried all the way home and needed herbal tea and a warm bath to calm my frazzled nerves.

The next day I went to see my regular doctor whom I hadn't seen yet. He was my general practitioner and I'd known him for eighteen years. I told him the news and he tightened up his face and looked at his paperwork while speaking.

'Well, you're going to terminate, right? I mean it would be the smart thing to do!' I was so devastated by his words I almost started crying.

'I haven't really decided anything,' I said. 'Why are you so against this pregnancy?' I asked him in a childlike way with such innocence in my voice I surprised myself.

'Well, the numbers add up, after all – your age and all. It's probably not going to be normal!' He kept looking at his papers. I wanted to hit him, to scream, to run. All I knew was this was all wrong. They were all wrong. I felt so protective of this little life inside that I was shocked and comforted by it at the same time.

A few days passed and I spoke to my closest relative back east on the phone. When I told her the surprising news she asked me what I planned to do. I told her I wanted to go through with the pregnancy. She hesitated at first and added, 'Haven't the experts been telling you what may happen? Aren't they advising that you terminate?' I told her what they said and she agreed with them all. 'Don't do this, please. Think about it again.'

Now I was sure this whole world was crazy and as unfeeling as a group of Nazis. There was nobody on my side; nobody who could see things my way. Maybe nothing would be wrong and this child would be fine in every way. There was still a chance all would go well and I would have a beautiful happy child that they all wanted to kill! I cried for what felt like days, holed up in my room, ignoring my two other children, both completely fine and perfect in every way.

Time seemed to go by quickly. I was beginning to show, my belly finally getting bigger, but nothing like my other pregnancies. I was now three-and-a-half months along; with my other children, I would have been as big as a horse by now. I was still wearing my regular clothes but feeling quite sickly on a daily basis, which reminded me that I was indeed with child. It was the first week of September and this was the time of most of my family's birthdays, so I was not thinking too much about the pregnancy, when the phone call came. I remember the nurse's voice and the words 'abnormal' and 'unusually low', but the rest is a blur. It was the call I dreaded and it was upon me. I asked her to please repeat herself and that's when she clearly stated, like she was reading a shopping list: 'Didn't they tell you that your test for the protein levels were really low, so your baby is most likely Downs?' I almost fell off the couch. I remember the phone dropping to the floor and her voice trailing off to a 'Hello? Hello?' and then she hung up and there was only my pain and the dial tone.

I have never in my lifetime felt such deep-seated grief. Not even when I miscarried a boy child at ten weeks, years earlier. Not even when my grandmother died after a very long and painful illness, did I feel this. I honestly felt like my guts were being ripped out from the inside. I started crying, heaving, sobbing so hard that my sides began to hurt. What a terrible thing to tell someone over the phone and in such a cold and detached way.

I cried uncontrollably for about 30 minutes and then my mind quickly went into 'nurse mode': must get information at once. Being a nurse for twenty-something years is hard to turn off and I was very thankful for all my expert training that made it possible for my mind to switch from devastation to information. I quickly ran to the bathroom, redid my makeup which was streaked black all over my face, and fixed my hair. I grabbed the car keys and raced to the local library which was two miles away. I grabbed every book I could find on Down syndrome, especially the ones that weren't over ten years old. I had no computer at home at this time, so I decided that books were the answer. Besides, you can really devour a book and you can't do that as well with an internet article. Books have always been a comfort to me. When I found out twenty-nine years ago that I had a debilitating disease called Crohn's, I stayed in my room and read eighteen books cover to cover about the disease. It comforted me to have knowledge of the subject before me. So, that's exactly what I did with this bit of disturbing information. I read and read about Down syndrome so that I was fully informed about every aspect of this new fact of my existence. I was so involved in gaining knowledge that I had little time for any more pity for myself. Actually, that was the last time I shed any tears about the baby until she was born. I knew in my heart that the chance of her having Down syndrome was very high, yet I chose to cling desperately to the small fraction of a chance that she might still be 'normal'. I guess it was my way of coping.

My biggest fear was the possibility that I wouldn't carry to term. Miscarriage was still a frightening reality for me. I started feeling movement and refused to get excited. I kept telling myself not to expect a birth and then I wouldn't be overly disappointed if I did miscarry. I still hadn't told anyone except my relative back east and my ex-husband. He was shocked, disturbed and somewhat aloof about the whole scenario. I mentioned that there could be a problem but he really didn't want to hear that. We agreed not to tell the kids in case I lost the baby.

After what felt like weeks but was in reality months, I had endured my grandfather's death, my oldest son's arrest and my youngest son's severe allergies. Christmas was upon us and I chose the family Christmas dinner to announce my pregnancy. Forks dropped to the fine china as quickly as the faces dropped and everyone was silent for a few minutes, which was a miracle in itself for my family. Finally my mother spoke. As she chose her words very carefully, she was trying hard not to look at me. 'I hope all goes well with this baby – thanks for telling us.' My two older children were not as gracious. My oldest son, who was home from his one-week stint in a county jail for driving under the influence, simply stated, 'Why? What were you thinking?' and shook his head as he shovelled another forkful of turkey to his mouth. My oldest daughter, a mother herself to two children, shook her head and said, 'Well, we are going to run out of room at the family table soon.' The emotion was so barren that I felt like I was dining with strangers. I went home and cuddled with my two youngest children as my 6-year-old son said to me, 'Momma, I love the baby and can't wait for her to come here, no matter what she's like.' I was so very thankful that one person on this planet was encouraging to me, and it happened to be my youngest child. I kissed his precious head and fell asleep holding him as he fell asleep holding me.

My legs started to swell, as well as my hands. It was January now, a new year and closer to the official 1 March 2003, due date.

My calculations were different. I believed my due date was 12 March. After all, I knew exactly when I had conceived the child. Movement of the baby slowed down a lot and I was very concerned. I was now on total bed rest and the worst was about to begin. My blood pressure kept going off the scale. On 13 February, I was rushed to hospital for probable pre-eclampsia, which can be fatal to mother and child. I stayed in the hospital all day and night. Early the next morning I left for home, with the promise to return the following day when they would begin inducing my labor. Upon leaving the hospital I went directly to our local drugstore and bought Valentine's Day gifts and cards for everyone, including all my children, and a cute stuffed pink bear wearing a stitched heart for my baby. I gave out all the gifts in case I didn't make it through. For the first time I was thinking that maybe I wouldn't survive the whole ordeal.

I went back to the hospital the next day, bags packed for me and a few things for the baby to come home with. I checked in and before long they started a oxytocin drip to induce my labor. My blood pressure was still high and my feet and wrists swollen. I watched the fetal monitor which was strapped to my belly and her heartbeat was nice and normal. As the contractions started, all that changed. Her heart rate dropped drastically with each contraction. I kept asking the nurse why this was happening. Finally they stopped the drip used to induce labor, and her heartbeat went back to normal. This went on all day Saturday and early Sunday. Finally by Sunday night the doctor on call for my obstetrician came in to tell me we were holding off on the inducement until my doctor came on duty in the morning. I slept restfully knowing all would finally be all right.

Early Monday, my doctor came into the room and said the contractions were adversely affecting the baby's heart so we could not go on with the labor. I thought he meant we would wait a few days and then see what happens. No – he made plans for an emergency c-section to be done in a few hours. I called my ex on the phone to tell him. He raced over after dropping the kids at my mum's and looked very grim and concerned. I was trying to stay optimistic. It was hard. I had ice chips and then they gave me some medicine to relax me. Before long they were shaving my stomach and prepping me for a spinal block.

At 2:13 pm on Monday, 17 February 2003, my baby, Layiah Vitina Wakan Cook, was born. I named her for all our mixed ethnicities: Layiah is Swahili, to honour her father's side of the family which is African American. It means 'born at night' – I felt after all she'd been through it was like being in the dark. Vitina, my Sicilian family name, means 'life' or 'little life'; my family has four generations of women with this name. Wakan is her Native American name which she shares with her older sister, again to honour her father's side who also have Cherokee nation in their blood. It is a name the Lakota nation gives to their spirit gods – it means 'courage' and 'strength'. I felt by honoring all the peoples that made up Layiah, they would surely protect her.

I barely got a chance to see her darling newborn face, as the nurses quickly suctioned, cleaned and whisked her away to the neonatal intensive care unit. I was frantic and wanted to know what was going on. All my ex kept doing was repeatedly questioning why they were saying she was probably Down syndrome. I had no time for him and all I cared about, as I lay on the table while they stitched me up, was what was happening with my child. Finally, after my loud protests, a nurse came by to tell me the baby was being taken to intensive care because she was under five pounds. Under five pounds! I was aghast! All my children were hefty eight-pound babies and never needed to be in an intensive care unit. I started to think the worst as they wheeled me into the recovery room. There I lay by myself, not feeling my legs due to the spinal block they gave me, wondering if I would ever get to hold my baby, the very baby that everyone told me not to have. This beautiful fragile little bird that nobody wanted me to bring into the world except a tender-hearted 6-year-old boy.

Tears began to stream down my face as I lay there wondering if they all were right. Maybe I never should have gone through with this. But the words of my grandfather kept ringing in my ears louder than my self-pity and my doubts. 'We come from strong people. Our people have survived much strife and pain. We have won all the wars that we fought and always came out victorious. We come from warriors, conquerors, conquistadors. We are always victorious. We are strong.' It sounded like a battle cry of the elders but for whatever reason, I suddenly had much faith in my bloodline. I felt as if my grandfather had sat down beside me to remind me of this. I think he was there. I felt stronger rather quickly and asked the nurse who came in to check me, if I could please see my child. She answered that they were taking measurements and doing tests with her and I would be able to see her soon.

It then dawned on me, she has made it! She has come through this whole pregnancy, she has been born into this world and she has breath in her lungs. She would be fine. I closed my eyes and knew that if she made it this far she was here to stay. A warrior. A survivor.

By 6 pm, I was wheeling myself in a wheelchair into the neonatal intensive care unit and saw my baby in an incubator with tubes and wires everywhere. I suppose most would have gasped at the sight, but I smiled, looking at my victorious one lying there like a little warrior. I got to hold her and smell her sweetness and feel her tenderness against me. I was tearing up with gratitude for this little one, for all her strength, all her courage. I felt very small holding one so big in spirit. Layiah Vitina Wakan was a fighter and I knew her life would be victorious. I knew this even when they told me she had two severe heart defects. I knew this when I was told she tested positive for trisomy 21 – Down syndrome. I knew this when she was undergoing open heart surgery and recovered in remarkable time. I knew this when I held her strong little hands in my fingers and looked into those determined eyes. And, I knew this today as I watched her turn 2.

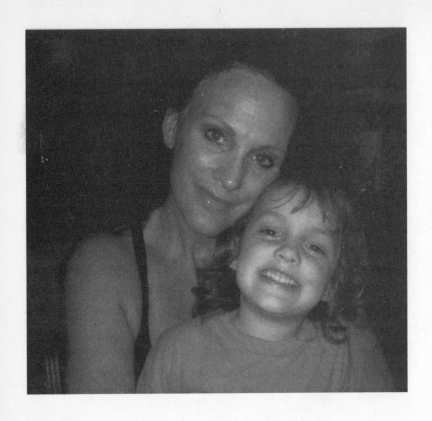

Diana D. Aldrich

Diana D. Aldrich lives in Portland, Maine, USA. Raised in her mother's dance studio, she developed an early passion for dancing and has performed and taught most of her life. She describes herself as 'a sucker for kittens' and now has twelve cats.

Diana D. Aldrich

ALL IS RIGHT WITH MY WORLD

You have to know the circumstances leading up to my pregnancy at 45, to be able to fully appreciate the way I felt as I was being deluged with negative comments, from my (former) obstetrician to the freakin' mailman – everyone had an opinion, and they were primarily negative!

I had divorced and remarried at 41 to a much younger man who had no children. Mine were 14 and 8 at the time. The deal was to try and have a biological one of our own, and if that didn't happen after a year, we would adopt. Funny, but when I told others of my plan to adopt, they didn't bat an eyelid; I guess it was okay to mother at an older age, but being pregnant at an older age was forbidden.

I was fortunate enough to conceive on our honeymoon, and had an uneventful pregnancy and delivery (c-section, like my previous two) that resulted in a ten-pound healthy daughter. We were all thrilled and, although most people agreed that it was 'better you than me' (as they put it – how I hate that phrase), they cut me some slack because my new husband now had his 'own' child.

We decided not to use any birth control to see if lightning would strike twice, but told no one about this decision – we knew what we would be up against. However I did mention to my new obstetrician what we were trying to do. Big mistake – huge. His response, and I quote: 'At *your* age, we should be talking menopause, *not* pregnancy – don't you agree?' No, I did not. I left his office, never to return. (Years later, when I delivered at the age of 46, I sent him a birth announcement, suggesting it was not too late for him to become a plumber.)

In the meantime my mother, who had been fighting a losing battle against Alzheimer's, moved in with us. For almost two years until her death, we cared for her at home. I am sure the stress did nothing to help my chances of conceiving, and month after month I was disappointed each time my period showed up – although now with less regularity as peri-menopause was settling in.

We lost her in November 1999. That Christmas I took my whole brood to Disney World for ten days to just relax and enjoy each other and the start of the new millennium – it had been a long two years for us all. We had a blast! I had finally (almost) given up on the chance of conceiving again as I knew that without medical assistance (i.e. donor eggs, in-vitro) my chances were like 0.02 percent or something.

Two weeks after getting home I still felt jetlagged and one of my fellow teachers joked: 'maybe you're pregnant.' I waited another few days for my period to start, and then bought a pregnancy test. I was so self-conscious at the drugstore – after all, I was now approaching 50! I took the test secretly in the bathroom as my family watched *Austin Powers*. Those two blue lines popped up in a nano-second; I was in shock. I motioned to my husband to follow me upstairs, where I relayed the news – he was so thrilled (and proud of himself). I was, too, but somewhat apprehensive because of my age and the accompanying horror stories I had always heard.

Now I had to find an obstetrician. But not just any obstetrician – a supportive 'this-is-great' obstetrician. I called a practice where the doctor had been around for years, hoping that he had seen it all, and I was lucky. He remembered a time before birth control pills, when everyone had a later-in-life baby, some after menopause. His own mother had had her last at 47, back in the 1930s. Terrific. Now for the rest of the planet . . .

We told no one until I was almost at the end of my first trimester and an early ultrasound confirmed an in utero viable fetus. I should have just said to people I was gaining weight during menopause – yikes! It just amazed me that people felt they could make such rude comments to a pregnant woman. In the background, always lurking, was the unspoken 'there will be something physically/mentally wrong with your child.' I could see it in their eyes; hear it in their tone of voice. Some actually voiced this to me, and asked if I would abort a Down's child.

The final straw came when I got the results of my AFP, which my obstetrician said would be way out of whack due to my age, so he was not going to pay too much attention to them. He only did the test to see about the neurological implications, and there were none, thank God. For my age, the chance of any complications was 1/33 – I'd take those odds to Vegas any day! My AFP came back 1/10; you could have heard a pin drop. Although there was still a 90 percent chance nothing was wrong with my baby, the looks on everyone's faces said it all, from the nurse to the radiologist, even to my obstetrician.

My obstetrician said that he would not insist on an amniocentesis unless the results of an in-depth ultrasound he was going to do indicated otherwise. The radiologist freaked – he said he wanted to go on record as not agreeing with this course of action, and that I was being 'stubborn, unreasonable and possibly doing harm to my baby' by refusing to acknowledge that something was probably very wrong. (I found out from a nurse later that the radiologist thought 'old women' such as myself were selfish and crazy to have children, and nature did not intend for it.) I asked this nurse what she thought. She said it would not be her choice, but that she knew why I was doing it, and she respected me for it.

Why couldn't everyone just act that way?

But that, unfortunately, was not the general consensus. I was thought of as totally selfish for not 'finding out' if my baby was 'perfect' or not. I had spent most of this pregnancy not enjoying it, but defending my right to have it, and have it the way I wanted it. I finally ended up being just as rude as those who were condemning me. When one acquaintance cornered me in the post office and told me that if she found herself pregnant at 46 she would 'kill herself', I asked her why not do us all a favour and kill herself anyway?

Well, to paraphrase an old saying, delivering well is the best revenge and that I did! A beautiful, wild, healthy daughter, Logan Alexandria (named for an X-Men character and her father's favourite Egyptian city). She continues to fascinate, challenge, exasperate and delight us all – and when I get those withering looks as my (older) friends and family watch me buckle up her safety belt or race off to ballet with her – as they pour yet another drink and whine for grandkids – I know that all is right with my world.

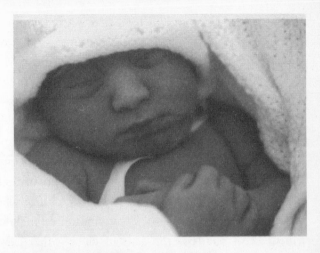

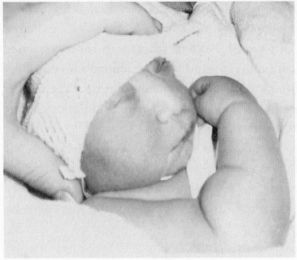

Teresa Streckfuss

Teresa Streckfuss lives in central Victoria, Australia, with her husband Mark and surviving children Cecilia, Sebastian and Elijah. With her husband, she is building a mud-brick house on six beautiful acres.

Teresa Streckfuss

IT'S ABOUT LOVE

This story really begins in 1996, nearly five years before Benedict's birth, when my sister and her husband discovered at their 18-week ultrasound that their first child was going to die. Thomas Walter had anencephaly, a neural tube defect where the top of the spinal column fails to close. Such babies are often stillborn. And while the condition is always fatal, some live for hours, days, sometimes even weeks after birth.

We were all so shocked. Nothing like this had ever happened in our family. Clare and Tom, newly wed and filled with the joy of starting a family together, had to suddenly adjust to the crushing news that their firstborn was so sick he would die shortly after birth, and there was nothing that could be done to save him. What were they to do? Their doctor falsely assured them that even Catholics were 'allowed' to have abortions after this diagnosis. But they believed life was precious and decided to carry Thomas Walter to term – to cherish him for the short time he would be with them.

So just before Christmas 1996, Thomas Walter came into the world. He lived for 17 hours. I will never forget holding my tiny nephew and marvelling at his chubby, beautifully formed hands. Apart from the top of his head, Thomas Walter was so perfectly formed, I remember wondering, 'Surely there's something they can do? Some kind of surgery? Anything?'

Mark and I married in February 1997. We planned on a big family, and I quickly became pregnant. I was very nervous when we had the ultrasound. I filled in the form with 'family history of neural tube defect'. I agonised over whether my baby's spine looked right. Fortunately, everything was fine and I gave birth to a healthy baby girl, Cecilia. Just over two years later, and following a miscarriage, Sebastian was born.

Our third child was due 17 July 2001. Leading up to the 18-week ultrasound, I found myself feeling very uneasy. I hadn't really felt any movement, which was odd, because I had felt Sebastian's first kicks very early. I now believe I subconsciously knew something was wrong. Generally, I am not a worrier, but I just couldn't shake this feeling of uneasiness. I had measured twelve weeks instead of thirteen at my first hospital appointment. I caught myself imagining that I was on the phone to Clare saying, '*It's happened to us, too!*' I asked myself – why am I thinking this? Then, the day before the ultrasound, I had my monthly midwives' clinic visit and the midwife let me listen to the baby's heartbeat. I was so relieved! So the next day – Valentine's Day – it was with no fear that we awaited our first look at our baby.

The appointment didn't start well. We left home in a rush that morning and forgot the appointment slip. The sonographer was hesitant to do the scan without it. I felt so disappointed. Eventually she agreed to perform the scan on the condition that we bring the form in after the scan. I felt so excited as I lay on the bed and she began to scan my belly. After all, I knew my baby was alive. I'd heard the heartbeat only yesterday, what could have happened since then?

As she began to scan she showed us that the placenta was lying across the 'os' or opening of the cervix – 'possible placenta previa' – meaning that I might need a caesarean. She explained that this was not necessarily a problem; depending on how the uterus stretched, the placenta may no longer be covering the 'os' at term.

Then she began to look at the baby. She became very quiet. She half-heartedly pointed out the feet, but didn't really say much at all. I thought this was odd, because she had been so chatty about the placenta. After a few minutes, she said she was very sorry but Mark would have to go home now and get the form, saying, 'I just need to check if the doctor wrote anything particular on it.'

I waited for over half an hour for Mark; it was a very long half hour. The sonographer kept coming in to see if he was back yet; she said something like, 'I just have to get someone else to check my pictures, no need to panic you just yet . . .' I wondered what she had seen, what was I supposed to be not panicking about? The screen was not really facing me properly, but I had seen her going over and over the baby's face. 'What is it? Doesn't my baby have a nose or something?' But deeper down my body seemed to be chanting, '*Anencephaly . . . anencephaly . . . anencephaly . . .*' Then I remembered what it said on the ultrasound slip: 'Check for congenital abnormality.'

When Mark returned we went back into the room with the sonographer and her superior. She showed him the placenta and he repeated a similar explanation to the one she gave us. He then took some of his own measurements. Eventually he turned to us and said, 'Now, there is a problem with the . . . *foetus*. We'll get someone down from Obstetrics to explain it all to you, and perhaps it's best if you save your questions until then.' I knew from his pause that he would have said *baby* if there had been nothing wrong. I wish I had just said, 'Is it anencephaly?' but instead I cried and let them lead us to the room where we were to wait.

This room was very, very cold, or perhaps it was we who were cold from shock. I kept saying to Mark, 'It doesn't have to be fatal. It could be anything – a heart problem, or kidneys, or lungs?' We waited for over 45 minutes for someone to come and tell us what was wrong. I can't describe the torture of that time. I began to play a little fantasy over in my mind: *The doctor would come in and say, 'I'm sorry, but your baby has Down syndrome,' and I would reply, 'Oh, that's okay! I thought you were going to say that our baby was going to DIE!' Then I would pick up my bag and we would go off to our planned Valentine's Day lunch.*

When she finally came in, the doctor sat down and asked if we had been told what was wrong. We said no, and she began to explain. 'There is a problem with the baby's skull.' I gasped and buried my face in my hands. So many images flashed though my mind – Thomas Walter squeezing my finger as I held him; his funeral; seeing his tiny coffin lowered into the grave; hugging my sister; *knowing* it would never be me burying a baby; *knowing* I didn't have Clare's strength.

Mark said, 'Do you mean anencephaly?' She said yes, and then asked what we knew about it. Mark explained about Thomas Walter. She asked a few questions and then told us that there were two options. We could continue on with the pregnancy, or we could terminate. Through my tears I said, 'No, we wouldn't do that.' It was very clear to us. There was no 'choice' other than to love our child. There was no easy way out; nothing could 'fix' our situation. Our baby would die, but it would not be by our hands. It was heartbreaking, but all our baby needed was love and we could give him that.

When we arrived home, Cecilia, now three years old, asked 'Are you a bit sad, Mama?' I replied, 'Yes, our baby's a bit sick – he has a sore head', then she gave me a cuddle. I wondered how we were going to explain to her that our much-looked-forward-to baby was going to die.

The two or three weeks after the diagnosis were by far the worst. I have no clear memory of this time, those weeks were a blur. I cried and cried. I also read. The 'carried to term' stories on the internet were amazingly helpful. I gathered so many ideas and so much encouragement. I found these stories so sad, yet so very uplifting. They portrayed the beauty of these babies' lives – no matter how short.

We hadn't been told the sex of our baby at that first ultrasound, so we arranged to have another one. We also had the second scan video-taped. We searched our baby names books for a name we liked which also had a nice meaning. When the sonographer told us we were having a boy, I felt so happy to know that I was carrying Benedict (meaning 'blessed') Oliver (meaning 'peace').

After the initial shock wore off, the rest of the pregnancy wasn't as bad as I'd imagined. Of course, it was all bittersweet. But getting to know Benedict – making things for him, giving him the life he was meant to have – was an honour. Losing him was the tragedy; to know we would lose him and still carry him was a gift. It was a gift of time and the opportunity to prepare for his short life after birth.

We made up a little baby announcement which said, *Mark and Teresa Streckfuss have been blessed with a new baby boy, Benedict Oliver. He is due on the 17th of July, 2001. A precious brother for Cecilia and Sebastian. Please pray for us as he has anencephaly and will not be with us long.* We sent this out to family and friends in the month after diagnosis. It was very important to me that Benedict was not forgotten; I didn't want people to just pretend that I'd never been pregnant.

Immediately after diagnosis I thought that the next four and a half months would be an unbearably long time. How could I possibly live through this whole experience? However, I was kept busy with all the plans and arrangements we were making, and looking back now it seems like no time at all. We had monthly midwives' clinic visits to start with. Our midwife, Maggie, was wonderful. Right from the start she was willing to do whatever we felt would help us in our preparation for Benedict's birth and death. She offered to have us come in every week, just to hear Benedict's heartbeat, if we wanted. She was so willing to help in whatever way she could. She admitted that she had never been in this position before and that she wanted to take the lead from us.

We had an overwhelmingly good response from all the medical staff – except one. He was a junior doctor working at the hospital, so fortunately we didn't run across him very often. But almost every time we did, he said something stupid. Our first encounter with him was the first time I was in hospital with previa. He was supposed to explain the condition to us, which he did – leaving us with the impression that it was no big deal because my baby wasn't 'viable' anyway. He said that if I was to haemorrhage the baby could bleed to death through the placenta but there was no real danger to me. This is not true, as I later learned. Another time I rang the hospital as I was having a bleed, and had to speak to him. After establishing that I was the woman with the 'anencephalic pregnancy', he made comments along the lines of, 'Since your baby's not viable, we won't worry too much, otherwise we'd be panicking. I suppose you might as well come into the hospital . . .' Apart from being hurtful, these comments were medically inaccurate as it was very important for my health that I go to the hospital as soon as I had any bleeding.

He also didn't even bother to read my birth plan because in his mind Benedict was just a 'non-viable foetus', and for some strange reason beyond his superior doctor's understanding, we did not choose to 'terminate' him when we found out.

It turned out that I did have grade IV placenta previa. This caused several small bleeds requiring short hospital stays for observation. I was in hospital seven times between weeks 28 and 36. This meant I had come into contact with most of the maternity staff before Benedict was born. At the hospital,

Benedict acquired quite a reputation for hiding from the sonic aide. Every time they would try to find his heartbeat there would be a flurry of kicking and he would just disappear! It often took them several minutes to track him down again. Maggie used to joke that he was hiding in 'the back room' – a kind of secret compartment. In some ways I didn't mind being in hospital all those times because three times a day I would get to hear his heartbeat and feel all those beautiful kicks as he tried to hide.

Because of the placenta completely covering the opening of the cervix, I had to have a caesarean section at 37 weeks. This suited me. I had read statistics that babies with anencephaly born vaginally have a higher chance of being stillborn. I couldn't imagine facing labour with the thought that Benedict could be stillborn. I wanted to say 'Hello' before 'Goodbye', and to me the only way of ensuring that was to have a caesarean. It was very important to us that Benedict be born alive.

On Monday 25 June, at 1:52 pm, Benedict Oliver was born. He lived for 24 hours and 13 minutes, dying at 2:05 pm on Tuesday. Unfortunately, Dr Tactless was on duty again when our beautiful boy died. He came bursting into our room and listened for Benedict's heartbeat and said, 'Okay, that's all fine,' before awkwardly leaving us again. Lucky he left. If he hadn't I might have screamed, 'THAT'S ALL FINE? THAT'S ALL FINE? GET OUT OF MY ROOM! MY BABY HAS JUST DIED! IT'S NOT ALL FINE! WHAT DO YOU MEAN, THAT'S ALL FINE?' I know what he meant. Our 'non-viable foetus' had died, as expected. He failed to recognise that we had just lost a person, someone we loved. The fact that we knew he would die and accepted this did not make it any less of a loss.

I don't think I can possibly tell you how beautiful Benedict was, or how sweet he smelled, or how much I wish those hours were frozen in time. He was so alive! He cried out, made facial expressions, wriggled. It was hard being all pinned down while they stitched me up. I couldn't hold him at first; because I had an IV drip in each arm, both were strapped down in a crucifixion position. Mark and our midwife held him on my chest near my face until I was stitched up and didn't need both IVs any more. I was so afraid he would die before I could hold and see him properly. I kept saying, 'Is he breathing?' and the midwife replied, 'He's struggling.' I asked if they needed to suction his airways, and she said, 'Yes, I think we'd better.' I wonder if they would have done that if I hadn't asked them? He was off being suctioned for a few minutes, and that was the only time he was ever out of our arms. He wore the tiny little premmie hat the hospital gave us. I had thought it would be too small, but it fit perfectly. His face was so sweet; he looked just like our other children at birth. He was just perfect. He weighed only 5 lb 9 oz (2600 grams) but he was very chubby and measured 46 cm long. He cried out at birth and several other times during his life – not a loud, healthy baby scream, but a cry nonetheless. He cooed, and made a soft little *pah-pah* noise when he breathed. He had light brown hair, ticklish feet, and once he sucked his thumb for about 15 minutes. We took so many photos. The time we had with him was so precious. We marvelled at how perfect he was, his soft cheeks, his feet and hands, and his sweet little face. I have never smelled such a sweet scent as the smell of his skin.

We had arranged for a priest friend to be present at Benedict's birth. As soon as he was born, Fr Colin was there to baptise and confirm him. Fr Colin gave us great support. He met with us while I was pregnant and gave me a special blessing and went through all the arrangements with us. Then after Benedict was actually born and he had finished his priestly duties, he grabbed the camera and started acting as photographer.

The theatre staff were wonderful – some of them cried, some

prayed, many of them patted my head or my hands while Benedict was being born. I remember the anaesthetist saying, 'He's a little saint already now, isn't he? He's been baptised and confirmed – he's perfect.' The midwives were beautiful. They left us alone as much as they could, popping in only when they had to. They were so caring. Benedict wasn't able to breastfeed, so they helped me express colostrum which we fed to him on a spoon. He had three feeds in his life this way. I don't think he ever got hungry, but I was glad I was able to nourish him this way. A few days after he died, when my milk came in, I wished he had lived long enough to have a proper feed, but at least he had something from me.

I have nothing but praise for the midwives and nurses who looked after us during Benedict's life before and after birth. They looked after Benedict with such love, and with the respect he deserved. Maggie, the midwife we saw for our antenatal visits, was particularly wonderful. She was with us at the caesarean, even though she was not on duty. She also came to Benedict's funeral, with one of the other midwives.

Benedict had lots of visitors. He met Cecilia and Sebastian, both sets of grandparents, aunties and uncles, cousins, his god-mother, and another priest friend. After about 10 pm we had him to ourselves. It was so nice to have the time that was left with just the three of us. We were so very, very tired, but we didn't want to sleep; we didn't want to miss what time we had left with him. I kept making little goals for him: *Please make it to midnight; please make it to 17 hours* (which was how long Thomas Walter lived), *please make it to morning*. I was so proud of him living as long as he did; I wanted to be able to say that he lived for a day. Eventually we were so exhausted that we took turns dozing, although I woke every time he moved. We both sang to him and Mark read to him, but mainly we just held him and loved him.

He started having short seizures on Tuesday morning, so we

knew his body was beginning to shut down. It was painful to watch, but we held him, stroked him, soothed him. He was very peaceful in between; the seizures only lasted a few moments each and came about one per hour. He died at 2:05 pm, just over 24 hours after he was born. After he died we bathed and dressed him. We kept his body with us overnight, and until the funeral director came to get him on Wednesday afternoon.

The night before his funeral, we took Benedict's body home and our families came over to say goodbye. I was worried how this would affect Cecilia and Sebastian, but it was really great for them. The times they saw him in the hospital were too short and with too many distractions. We have some beautiful video footage of Sebby vigorously rocking Benedict in the cradle saying, 'Bay-beee, bay-beee, bay-beee'. Cecilia sang to him in the morning, and made sure he had his teddies with him. These toys are looked after with extra care now because they are 'Benedict's Teddies'.

He spent the night in the cradle by our bed, and in the morning I dressed him in the outfit I'd bought to bury him in. It was very hard to wrap him up for the last time and put him in the coffin. It was even harder to close the lid and know that I would never see his sweet face again. He was snuggled up in a cosy red polar fleece blanket I made for him. We drove him to the church. It was very sad to think that was the only time all five of us would be travelling together.

We had been grieving over Benedict for four months already, so the funeral was not as intense as we anticipated. Naturally I was sad, but not hysterical like I thought I would be. Benedict is now buried beside Thomas Walter at the small cemetery near where we live. It is very sad to go to the cemetery and see his tiny little grave, but I am glad he is next to his cousin.

You may wonder at me referring to Benedict as 'beautiful' and 'perfect' when he had anencephaly, which is an obvious physical defect, but he was beautiful and perfect and every other cute baby description you could think of – *he was my son!* I don't love Cecilia and Sebastian because they're healthy; I love them because they are my children. I miss him so much, but I wouldn't trade his life for anything. And while this has been the most painful experience I've ever had to endure, it's probably been the most beautiful as well. Benedict spent his whole life in the arms of people who loved him; who could ask for a better life?

It didn't take us long to want another baby. My caesarean had been a 'classical incision' rather than the safer 'lateral incision', so we were distressed to learn that I would only be allowed to deliver by caesarean from now on; the risks of uterine rupture during labour were considered too high. I conceived again six months after Benedict was born. Dosed up to the eyeballs with folic acid, I was pretty confident of a healthy baby. I was offered a scan at my 12-week appointment and agreed. There was my baby, perfectly formed – but still. The obstetrician was very nice, he gently told me that he should be seeing a heartbeat or some movement. I looked at the screen, silently pleading with my baby: 'Just kick, please just kick . . .' But she had already gone, just a day or two before.

Having some understanding of loss and grieving after losing Benedict helped us cope with the loss of this baby. We named her Hannah, and made up a booklet of what little memories we had of her. I felt as if we were creating a space in the timeline of our family that was just Hannah's, and would always be just hers, and then it was okay to move on. I've never felt that way about my first miscarriage (my second pregnancy). We didn't stop to allow a special place for that child – we didn't know how to grieve then.

Three months after losing Hannah we felt ready to conceive again. After a nerve-wracking although uneventful pregnancy, Elijah was born in January 2003. It was such a relief to finally hold him in my arms. We felt like first-time parents again; it was such a change to actually bring our baby home and watch him grow; we marvel at everything he does. Knowing that life can be so brief has enabled us not to overlook one tiny bit.

We knew we would not feel ready for another pregnancy for a long time after Elijah. The two caesareans, which had both been classical, were eighteen months apart, so there were physical reasons for me – as well as psychological ones. The worry over anencephaly and miscarriage, the physical fatigue involved in pregnancy, the daily injections (due to a blood-clotting disorder) were all substantial reasons for us to enjoy Elijah and postpone any thought of pregnancy.

However, when Elijah was just nine months old, I found myself pregnant again – the first 'surprise' pregnancy we'd had. The mental unpreparedness far outweighed the physical. It wasn't coping with another baby that worried me – it was the pregnancy itself. This new baby would arrive just a week before Benedict's third birthday and anniversary. The anxiety was unbearable. We looked forward to the 12-week ultrasound to put our minds at ease. Of course our baby would be okay . . .

As luck would have it, we had the same ultrasound technician who diagnosed Benedict. As soon as she turned on the scan I could tell the baby had anencephaly. Even though I told myself I could be wrong, I could see the head was much too small. My heart raced as I waited. 'What neural tube defect was it last time?' she asked. When we replied 'Anencephaly,' she said, 'I'm sorry, but it looks like the same thing again. Unfortunately we can't diagnose these things any earlier.' I thought, 'Earlier?' Twelve weeks was far too early if you asked me. But then it dawned on me – she thought we were going to have an abortion. I said, 'I carried our son to term, and that's what I'll be doing again.' We didn't let ourselves fall apart until we got to the car.

Just when we were getting used to the idea of me being pregnant again, we had to adjust our plans, this time to include the knowledge that we were going to lose another baby.

I was still afraid of miscarriage, as I didn't feel any movement until around 20 weeks. My GP informed me that the scan had also picked up a low-lying placenta. Twelve weeks is far too early to diagnose placenta previa, but with my history of two classical caesarean scars and previous placenta previa it was a pretty high risk. I looked up 'placenta accreta' on the internet and found that I had a 47 percent chance of developing the condition. Placenta accreta is a complication where the placenta attaches deep into the uterine muscle instead of just on the surface of the uterus. It almost always necessitates a hysterectomy. I felt like I had far too much on my plate.

I couldn't help comparing everything to Benedict. As we felt that everything went perfectly with Benedict's delivery and life, we worried that this time things could only be worse. This baby couldn't live as long as Benedict; my caesarean couldn't be without complication. Distinguishing this baby mentally from Benedict was almost impossible, after all, his was an earth-moving, life-altering experience – it was not something we were supposed to have to do twice.

At eighteen weeks I had my first antenatal appointment after the diagnosis. I was sure the results would have been sent up to the antenatal section. But as I sat in the waiting room for 45 minutes, surrounded by happy pregnant women, I began to realise that the information hadn't been passed on to the staff. They would never have left me sitting there if they'd known. With a growing sense of dread, I realised I might have to break the news myself. A midwife finally called my name. As we walked to her room she asked me, 'How are you?' in the kind of way you do when you are sure the answer is, 'Fine!' I replied with a noncommittal, 'Not too bad . . .' I kept thinking, 'When she opens my file, then she'll know . . .' Unfortunately, as the consultation went on I could see that the scan results had not been forwarded on and I would have to say something. The midwife asked, 'Have you had a scan already?' To which I replied, 'Yes, at twelve weeks, and this baby has anencephaly.' She just looked at me for a moment, then she said, 'But you've already lost a baby to anencephaly! Oh, that's just too much for one person to bear!' She was very nice; she tried to comfort me – I had completely lost my composure by this stage. I asked if Maggie would be able to handle my antenatal visits again, as she had with Benedict's pregnancy, and although she told me Maggie wasn't working there any more, she promised to sort something out. I almost felt more sorry for her than I did for myself right then. I can't imagine how awful it was to be in that position, with no forewarning or time to prepare yourself.

Two weeks later she rang me at home to say that she had spoken to Maggie, who had readily agreed to do my antenatal visits, even though she only worked in delivery now. I felt an enormous weight lift off me. It was such a relief to know that Maggie would be caring for us again. She knew what to do, she knew us, she'd done this before, things would be all right.

That same week I had my second ultrasound and we were both pleased and saddened to hear we were having a girl. We had hoped for another daughter. After three boys in a row, we had begun to think that Cecilia would be our only daughter. It was hard to hear that it was a daughter who was not going to stay. But now we had a name, a beautiful name we had been waiting to use for a long time – Charlotte Mary.

Naming Charlotte gave her her own identity, distinct from her brother. She had quite a different personality from Benedict. She was very active in utero, whereas Benedict was quiet. Charlotte never minded the Doppler checking her heartbeat; Benedict hated it.

How do you do this twice? With Benedict's pregnancy we'd done it all; were we supposed to do all those things again? Two mizpah coins? Post out prayer requests all over again? If we did the same things over, were we cheating Charlotte? It took several weeks to sort through these feelings, and in the end find peace with a plan for Charlotte's journey.

Of course, I still had to deal with a lot of dark, out-of-control feelings. At times I felt like a lightning rod, just waiting for the next storm to break. While pregnant with Benedict, I never really asked, 'Why?' As my sister had lost a baby this way, it made more sense to ask 'Why not?' But to have this happen twice! My heart cried, 'Why, why, why?' Why couldn't it have been something she could live with? What could we be supposed to learn this time that couldn't have been learnt from Benedict? Why couldn't we have the big family we had always wanted? And the most frightening question of all – Would this happen again? Having had placenta previa before, I was living in expectation of the bleeding starting and wondering if this time I would haemorrhage and need an emergency caesarean. However I made it to 31 weeks before my first very small bleed. Going into hospital bleeding like that was like a painful déjà vu. An ultrasound confirmed grade III previa. I had two more hospital stays over the next few weeks. I had one last ultrasound at 36 weeks, and much to everyone's surprise, my placenta had moved up.

Now the likelihood of hysterectomy was small, and my anxiety about the caesarean was greatly reduced. I had been so afraid that if something was to go wrong with the surgery and I needed to be given a general anaesthetic, Charlotte could die while I was unconscious. I was so afraid of missing her time.

Thankfully my caesarean went unbelievably well. It took a long time to actually deliver Charlotte, because in that last week she had turned and was breech. It seemed to take forever and I was afraid that she had already died and they didn't know how to tell us. But eventually there was a little cry and there she was! Chubby and cute and covered in chunky vernix, and so much like Benedict.

Charlotte was held by my chest so I could see her. She looked so purple and still, I was really worried. I asked Maggie if she was breathing, and she said, 'I think I'll take her over here and rub her down.' She told me the next day that Charlotte's pulse had dropped and she thought she was going to die there in theatre, so she'd 'rubbed her down and given her a stern talking-to'. When she carried her back she was beginning to get nice and pink, and we were unaware of how close we had been to losing her then.

As soon as she was born, Fr Anthony, another young priest friend of ours, came in and baptised and confirmed her. He took many beautiful photos and some video too. These short snippets of video are so precious. We didn't know he was filming, so we were just getting to know Charlotte and it was very natural and unaffected. Fr Anthony stayed with me in recovery, and later completed the baptism ceremony back in our room. His presence was calming and uplifting and we were so grateful to him for being there for us at this time.

Charlotte met her siblings – our 4-year-old said, 'Oooh, she's so cute!' Our 6-year-old took a while to get used to her, but fortunately had enough time to fall in love with her sister before she died. Elijah, just 17 months old at the time, didn't seem to even notice there was a new baby in the room. Charlotte met cousins, aunts, uncles, grandparents, friends. She was so quiet and still, we were sure she wouldn't last as long as Benedict.

There were so many times over the six days she was with us when we thought she was going to die. The first was about 11 pm the first night. There was no way, we were sure, she would get two dates to her name. We were so wrong. There were at least three shifts of nurses who I informed, 'I don't think she's going to last very long now.' Every time I thought she was dying, I was able to appreciate how long we'd had her for. She was so lovely and pink, and sweeter than anything I've ever beheld. She was quiet and peaceful, and seemed so much smaller and more fragile than Benedict even though she weighed 6 lb 9 oz, a whole pound heavier than he was.

At the end of the second day we realised that we had spent the entire day waiting for her to die. We decided this was a bad way to be, and made a conscious effort to enjoy her life – rather than just wait and anticipate her death. We desperately needed some sleep, so my mother and sister came and sat with Charlotte for six hours on the second night, and Mark and I were able to rest. We were really hesitant about this. We didn't want anyone but the two of us with her when she died. On the other hand, we had to get some sleep. So we gave them instructions to wake us if anything happened.

Maggie was able to come back in on the second and third days and spend a few hours with Charlotte. She got to connect with Charlotte as a real person, not just as an idea. She gave Charlotte the cutest teddy. We wrapped her arm around it and she held it for the rest of her life.

Charlotte reacted to her surroundings much more than Benedict. Although we have no way of knowing how much higher brain function she had, she definitely had some degree of awareness. Charlotte reacted to the camera flash, she tracked light with her eyes, she startled at a loud noise, she had ticklish hands and feet, she clearly felt pain when the dressing on her head was moved, and was obviously more peaceful and comfortable after we had redone her dressing. And she got hungry. It took me a while to realise this. I didn't even consider the possibility of actually breastfeeding her. Several times she was fretting and making little crying noises and we didn't know what to do. Then she started to make this loud smacking noise, from sucking her tongue against her palate and I thought, 'Maybe she can suck?' When I tried to feed Charlotte she opened her mouth into exactly the right shape, she sucked and lapped the milk which I expressed into her mouth. She didn't actually latch on, but it was so beautiful to have her sucking and swallowing and enjoying real milk. As I hadn't yet weaned Elijah, I had enough milk to easily express into her mouth. When I would feed her she'd drink for up to an hour and then be peaceful and content again.

Because she lived for so long, we were able to observe her face changing (as with all newborns). Over the first 24 hours or so her nose straightened out and turned into the same nose our other children have. She was born with my dint in her chin, but after a few days she developed a very defiant chin, which is a Streckfuss characteristic. She would stick her chin out and pout her lips in the most adorable way. She got a little jaundiced on day three, but she had the sweetest rosy cheeks. Her ears were perfectly formed and she had lots of black hair at the back of her head.

Every day we'd have a moment when we'd think, 'This is it . . .' We held an oxygen tube in front of Charlotte's face from the second morning onwards. It wasn't life support and it didn't keep her alive, but I do think it kept her comfortable and helped her to pick up again after having a seizure. Then we got to day four and they started to talk about us going home. We had never even hoped for that. When it came time for us to go on Friday, we were afraid to leave the oxygen – 'What if she dies in the car without it?' Eventually the hospital arranged to send us home in an ambulance. I was so afraid she'd die on the way home, but she made it, and we had one beautiful night with her at home before she died.

When she died on Saturday, it was at home with both of us

there, holding her, loving her, and actually letting her go. After six wonderful, eventful days surrounded by our love and prayers, and those of our friends, family and thousands of strangers across the world, she left our arms for heaven. It was the 26th – Benedict's anniversary.

So, side by side our babies lie. Charlotte, Benedict and their cousin Thomas Walter, all in a row. The last two babies buried at this cemetery were both ours. It is sad, but there has been so much good, so much happiness, so many blessings mixed in with all the heartbreak. I am sad they couldn't stay, but I am so glad that they came at all. We have certainly experienced that peace which passes all understanding during this time. To have known and loved them is such a precious gift that we will hold in our hearts forever.

Some day we will have another baby. We hope and pray we will get to keep the next one. The risk of losing another child seems terrifyingly real to us, but one day we will find the courage to risk our hearts again.

Why carry a dying child? A mother's perspective

Many people have wondered, 'What's the point?' or perhaps pitied us for 'having' to continue carrying a child who is not going to live for long. I understand these thoughts, because when my sister was carrying Thomas Walter I really didn't properly comprehend the whole situation. I knew it was the 'right' thing to do. I didn't question that I would have no other option if the same thing ever happened to me (although I was sure it never would!). But I thought how awful it was to know for over four months that the child you are carrying is unable to live outside your womb.

Once he was born, I was able to hold my nephew and see him finally as a real person – a precious unique creation. It was then that I began to realise there was a lot more to it than mere 'ethics'.

When, much to my disbelief, my own baby, Benedict, was diagnosed with this same condition four years later – I was finally able to grasp it, although it has taken me a long time to be able to put my thoughts into words. It is only since Charlotte's diagnosis that I have found words that almost convey my feelings.

Some people think we carried Benedict and Charlotte to term because we don't agree with abortion, because we're Catholic, or perhaps because our nephew was carried to term after a fatal diagnosis. While these factors probably all played a part in our immediate refusal to 'terminate', this is not what it's all about. It's about love! It's about our babies! We do not possess more strength than other people. It's not because we can cope where others wouldn't. There is no way to avoid the sad fact that these babies cannot live long after birth with this condition, but causing them to die earlier will not stop this happening. Causing them to die earlier will only take from us the beautiful experience of knowing and loving them.

The tragedy is not the fact that we know our baby will die. The tragedy is that our baby will die. It is not nice to know for months beforehand, but it gives us a chance to appreciate a life so brief, and not to miss a moment.

The value of Thomas Walter, Benedict and Charlotte cannot be measured by the length of their lives – we don't apply this yardstick to adults, so why should we to babies? A baby is a gift, a new entity, a precious individual. We are created for a purpose, there is a reason for our being here. Even if that reason is unclear to us most of the time, we are constantly affecting other people in our families and communities. Who knows what purpose can be fulfilled in nine months and one day? I do know that Benedict left a lasting impression on our family. He made us slow down, savour life, and treasure our other children even more. He made us realise that we cannot control or predict what will happen in the future;

he made us rely on God.

So don't pity us for carrying a child we know will die. Carrying this beautiful person is an honour. Grieve for the fact that our baby will die. We wouldn't wish away the time we had with Benedict, or Charlotte, just to save us the pain of losing them. I've always thought of it like this: if your 3-year-old was diagnosed with fatal cancer and had only four months to live; would you prefer the doctor kill your child straight away so that you didn't have to wait for his/her impending death? Or would you prefer to spend as much time as you could with your child and love him/her for as long as you had left?

Someone asked us after Benedict died, 'Was it worth it?' Oh, yes! For the chance to hold him, and see him, and love him before letting him go. For the chance for our children to see that we would never stop loving them, regardless of their imperfections? For the chance to give him everything we could? Oh, yes! Love your children, and remember that they each have their own unique mission. Children are always and only a blessing, even if they don't stay very long.

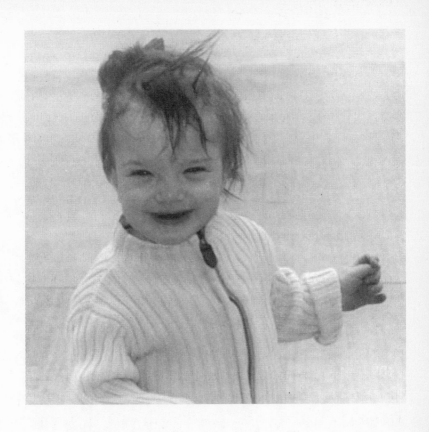

Sandi Seyferth

Sandi Seyferth lives in the Midwestern United States (Michigan) with her husband Patrick and their five children. She is a stay-at-home mom and enjoys managing her active family; volunteering at school and within the community; photography; scrapbooking; and travel. As a 'retired' certified public accountant, she hopes to one day assist her husband's busy law practice.

Sandi Seyferth

YOUR BABY WILL DIE: THE STORY OF GRACE

In early June 2002, my husband and I found out we were expecting our fifth child. We were very excited about the news and everything seemed normal as I began the familiar symptoms of nausea, moodiness and fatigue, and I silently prayed for an uneventful nine months.

During my first doctor's visit, the need for prenatal testing was brought up. I listened politely, but quickly informed him that I was really not interested and that I would be committed to the pregnancy regardless of any anomalies. He went on to explain that I really did not know what I would do if I had the information and I should get it anyway. Since I continually declined testing, the doctor wanted to make sure that my ultrasound was done right at 18 weeks.

The ultrasound date came quickly and my husband and I were excited to see our growing baby. The routine ultrasound seemed to be moving along okay, although it took a very long time and the technician seemed to be taking a lot of pictures of my baby's bones. We thought this was rather odd, and joked between ourselves with eye gestures and smiles. After all the ultrasound pictures were completed, the technician left and was gone for a long time. When she returned she began taking additional measurements of our baby's kidneys. I started to worry, but was somewhat relieved that we were not immediately referred to the staff doctor. After that, we were free to go home.

I phoned my doctor that afternoon and when he called me back he announced that there were some problems with my baby. My amniotic fluid was very low; my baby's bones were small; the femur bones were curved; the head was odd-shaped, and the kidneys, stomach and bladder were abnormally sized. In addition, the report said that my baby's left foot was turned – possibly clubbed. He referred me to a perinatologist – and added that the report indicated a pregnancy which, in his opinion, 'smelled like chromosomal problems', especially in light of my advanced maternal age (37) and that I should keep my options open.

My husband and I reacted quickly. We were lucky enough to get an appointment with the Director of Ultrasound who is a board-certified perinatologist at a well-regarded research facility in our major city. The hospital and our doctor both have national reputations in handling high-risk pregnancies. We were hopeful that the small local hospital that performed the first ultrasound was simply wrong and that the specialists here would set the record straight. My ultrasound was scheduled for Thursday 12 September.

Our world would never be the same after that day. After an hour-long ultrasound performed by a highly skilled technician, the nationally regarded perinatologist personally came in to perform a second ultrasound, in uncomfortable silence.

We watched in horror at the whispering between the growing team. Finally, the curved femurs were pointed out to my husband and me and we were then asked to wait for the doctor in the office down the hall. She arrived about half an hour later and informed us of the devastating diagnosis: a lethal type of skeletal dysplasia. As a result, there was no reason to mince words: 'Your baby will die.'

Lethal skeletal dysplasia, the doctor explained, is a rare form of dwarfism in which the child's arms and legs are extremely short and malformed, and the chest cavity is very small. In these circumstances, a baby cannot sustain life for more than a few hours because the narrow chest cavity does not allow the lungs to develop properly or to expand and provide the proper amount of oxygen necessary to sustain life. So long as the baby is attached to the mother, she will develop and grow. However, the cutting of the cord is itself the severing of the only lifeline sustaining the child. As a result, the baby dies of respiratory distress. The options: 'interruption' of the pregnancy, or continue on, with periodic monitoring of the baby's condition, and prepare for a burial shortly after the birth. We left in a pool of tears and shattered dreams.

Over the course of the next few days my husband and I discussed our so-called 'options'. We did not want to terminate, although we did not yet quite understand how long I should carry the baby – whether or not I should deliver early after seven months. We talked with friends and family. We had such a range of advice, however one thing really hit home. My sister-in-law's priest explained the confusing situation in clear and beautiful words: God does not value a life as a number of years (or even days) we've spent alive here on earth. 'All life is equally valuable, no matter how short, and we can never fully understand the impact of one life on all of humanity.'

We decided to carry our child to term and to love her for the time she would spend with us, inside me. As we made this decision, we embraced her sweet kicks each night; we found out the sex of our baby (something we had never done before) and named her Grace, which means 'undeserved gift from God'.

My original obstetrician, on receiving the ultrasound report and learning of my desires to carry the baby to term, quickly dropped my case. He did not want to handle my prenatal care and even said that 90 percent of people with my diagnosis would have 'made the appointment' by now. I transferred to the perinatal facility, which provided an entire team of specialists who would closely follow our case.

I entered a fetal assessment program and had ultrasounds performed monthly to monitor my baby's progress. Our meetings were coordinated by the Director of Genetics, who was not at all sensitive to my decision not to terminate. In fact, until 28 weeks had passed and a termination was no longer possible, this topic was the focus of our monthly meetings. My husband and I stayed the course of our decision and avoided the geneticist's attempts to spread doubt and fear. However, I must admit, it was very difficult not to be bothered by his comments and advice.

The diagnosis of our daughter's condition was 'validated' at each ultrasound: small femur bones (and other long bones); an easily manipulated bone structure; and a very narrow chest cavity. Her feet were always perplexing to the doctors; no one was ever quite sure what was wrong with them and this apparently was all part of the skeletal dysplasia. During one of the assessments, I had a three-dimensional ultrasound. A beautiful clear image of our daughter's face was given to us. We kept this image on our refrigerator door. It carried me through the tough times and helped me believe in this little life inside of me (although the General Electric commercials with the song 'The first time ever I saw your face' were simply too much to bear). I longed for the day I would hold her – even if her time alive was very short. I longed for her just the same.

The last of my six ultrasounds was performed on 30 December. Grace's measurements were so poor at this time that they stopped the ultrasound after measuring only one side of her body. In the exam room were the Director of Ultrasound, Director of Genetics, two neonatologists and a technician. They all agreed that the prognosis of lethal skeletal dysplasia was correct and would take Grace's life upon birth. We provided a birth plan which stated that there would be no ventilation, that the baby was to be wrapped in a blanket and given to my husband and me after birth so that we could spend time with her. Her predicted life span was given as four to six hours. The hospital agreed to let our four other children come to see their sibling. We made plans to have the baby baptised. The only other arrangements we made were with the cemetery.

On 8 January, 2003, I started to have some slight cramping and other symptoms indicating that I may be going into early labor. My husband had a short trip to Arizona planned and was leaving on the early flight the next day. I told him about my symptoms and he insisted I call my doctor, who said to come to the hospital in the morning and he could check me out. Convinced that I may be going into labor, I packed my bags and loaded them in the car.

On the morning of 9 January I was hooked up to a fetal monitor and checked for dilation/effacement at the hospital. The doctor calmly stated that I had not dilated at all and my cervix didn't appear shortened. He said he was confident I would not deliver until closer to my due date – 18 February. He told my husband to catch the next plane out. Relieved by the news, I drove my husband to the airport on an unusually warm and sunny January day. Feeling better than I had in months, I drove home and felt an unusual peace and happiness. Not that my daughter would live – but just that I could endure what lay ahead, although there were emotional lapses caused by such things as the expiry date on the carton of milk that was after the date my baby would be born and die.

At about 2 pm that day, I received a phone call from my husband. The fog was so bad in Phoenix they could not fly. He returned home. Incredibly, at about 11:30 that same evening, my water suddenly broke (at 35 weeks' gestation). We called my parents to come stay with the kids, and left for the hospital. Our adrenaline was high and our emotions ranged from fear, sadness, longing to finally hold our baby, and confusion. On arrival, my doctor examined me, checked the position of the baby via ultra-sound, ordered an epidural, and informed the nurse that there was no need for a fetal monitor. The doctors were so sure that Grace would not live that there was no need for monitoring.

Grace Marie was born at 11:19 am. All eyes were on my daughter as she emerged screaming from the womb – and my first impression was Wow! She doesn't look that unusual to me. Weighing in at 4 lbs 2 oz, Grace was indeed a small baby. Doctors and nurses immediately began to assess her breathing and vitals. There were about eight to ten medical doctors and nurses in the room assisting. In addition, several other resident doctors and researchers were in the doorway and hallway, hoping to catch a glimpse of the 'dysplasia baby'. Our nurse, who by this time had become completely empathetic to our situation, forced unnecessary observers away from our room.

The doctors and nurses were busy, yet no one was saying very much. They gave Grace a little oxygen to 'pink her up' and, given the fact that she was five-and-a-half weeks early, her respiratory wellness was no less than unbelievable. Grace's APGARs were eight and nine. They wrapped her in a blanket and handed her to my husband and me. We joyfully embraced Grace and took lots of pictures of her.

Grace was cleaned up and while she was gone my parents and our children arrived, followed by my two sisters-in-law. Then came the chaplain, who performed the most beautiful baptism of Grace right in our labor and delivery room. We were all crying and so happy that Grace was alive long enough to be baptised. We took pictures of everyone holding her. Despite the fact that we were still not expecting much more time with her, everyone was so happy. We were celebrating.

About an hour later, Grace began a form of respiratory distress known as 'grunting'. The neonatal nurse who had been staying with us since her birth needed to take her to the newborn intensive care unit for evaluation. We all feared that this was the beginning of the end for our beautiful daughter. The jovial mood in our room immediately changed to sadness. Our family left saying tearful goodbyes to Grace and we went out to talk to the neonatologists.

The neonatologists wanted to do a variety of tests on Grace right away. They informed us that a team of pediatric doctors were already waiting for her at the Children's Hospital – connected to the delivering hospital by underground tunnel. We agreed to have Grace tested. My husband went with her. During the tests, Grace screamed so loud he couldn't believe it was our little four-pound baby.

When they returned, the doctors took Grace back to Special Care and we waited anxiously for the results of the tests. About two hours later, the head of Neonatology called and asked if she could meet with us in our room. She excitedly told us the unbelievable news: the X-rays indicated that Grace did not have skeletal dysplasia (lethal or non-lethal) and that her bone structure was very proportionate. They felt she was small, however did not feel she was out of the normal range (she was in the tenth percentile for height and weight). The doctor also announced that Grace had oxygen saturation of 100 percent. Apparently the respiratory grunting had resolved itself when Grace screamed the mucus out of her lungs during testing. She was nippling bottles well, and maintaining her own temperature. They had no reason to even keep her in Special Care, and were bringing her down to 'room in'!

We were in a complete state of shock. My husband and I just hugged and cried. Family and friends were called and we cried with each one of them. Everyone was stunned by Grace and the amazing result after all the terrible predictions. My husband and

I spent the next two days in the hospital with Grace; we took turns just holding her, staring at her. We were so filled with happiness and thankfulness. The nurses had a baby shower to celebrate her life. On Sunday we were discharged together. The memorial service we had planned for Grace was immediately changed to a celebration of her life!

Grace is now fifteen months old and an exuberant bundle of energy. She is walking, talking and doing all the things a normal 15-month-old would do. She is still a tiny little thing – 16 pounds at one year of age – but it has not stopped her one bit. She is a light to our whole family and a constant reminder that you never can lose faith even when all seems hopeless. I shudder to think of my feelings on this day had we listened to the many specialists who felt 'interrupting' this pregnancy would be our best option. Would I ever have known the truth about my lovely daughter?

Even if the diagnosis had been correct, the hours or even minutes holding her would have been easily worth the pain and suffering. Later, many people told us that seeing me carry this baby had affected their lives in ways I would never know. We are forever grateful that we listened to our hearts.

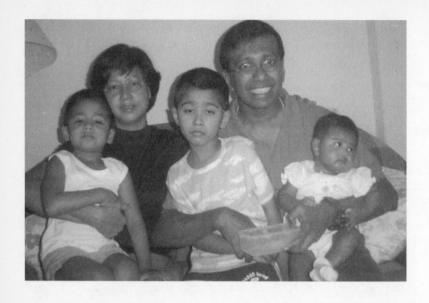

Nirmmala Jegathesan

Nirmmala Jegathesan lives in Singapore with her husband Jega and three children. No longer able to swing from tree to tree, Nirmmala now practises yoga instead. Should you pass by a small park in Central Tampines, Singapore, and see a tiny, middle-aged woman clinging valiantly to her lotus posture with a baby in a sling and a 3-year-old trying to disengage the centuries-old posture, it's probably her. She dedicates her story to Jega, who 'always held my hands when I faltered in my steps and assured me that "All will be well".'

Nirmmala Jegathesan

GIVING LIFE A CHANCE

We met late in our lives, Jega and I. I was then a 31-year-old youth co-ordinator with the Singapore Red Cross Society, while he was a 33-year-old flight steward with Singapore Airlines who wanted to get into the teaching profession. We came from somewhat different backgrounds. I had spent twenty-one years of my early life running bare-footed amongst squawking chickens and slinky cats in a rustic Malay village tucked away near the infamous Changi Prison where hundreds of captured allied forces were imprisoned and tortured by Japanese occupants during World War II. I lived with my three sisters and two brothers in an attap-roofed house built by our eccentric father who refused to install electricity in our home and saw the invention of the television as the ultimate evil of our times. It left all of us with ample time to pursue hobbies including reading, sports, fishing and literally swinging from tree to tree.

Jega grew up in an apartment with his aged grandparents along with eight uncles and their spouses. He rocked to the music of the Beatles and the Bee Gees with his younger sister and brother. He became passionate about reading, soccer and healthy eating.

Our first meeting took place at a food centre along East Coast Beach. It was arranged by two persistent mutual friends who felt sure that we were made for each other. What utter nonsense, I thought. I had long given up on fairy tales and the Mills & Boon romance novels of my teenage years. But it was love at first sight for both of us.

We discovered that we had so much in common: we shook our heads at loud techno music and smiled at stray dogs chewing on bones at the food stalls. We also discovered that we preferred the Ferris wheel to the roller-coaster ride – the former was more predictable. We also believed passionately that children are the real teachers – they teach lessons no one else can to the adult human hearts. And like everyone else who lived to see their long-awaited dreams come true, we couldn't wait to spend the rest of our lives together, and got married a year later. We also knew that we wanted children as soon as they would come to complete our little family unit.

I gave birth to our first child, Seth, a year into our marriage. It was an easy pregnancy until suddenly from 28 weeks for two-and-a-half months he stopped growing in my womb and I started experiencing a series of early contractions. This was attributed to the presence of anti-nuclear antibodies (ANA) in my blood, which the physician explained could cause premature births. I was given a series of steroid injections to boost his growth and he was delivered via caesarean section at 38 weeks.

During my teenage years, I had developed a 'butterfly rash', a classic sign of lupus, an auto-immune illness in which the body produces antibodies and attacks its own healthy cells. But I did not carry the other symptoms such as organ involvement and extreme fatigue. The rash faded away with the daily use of sun-screen and I happily ignored the presence of anti-nuclear antibodies in my blood as my lupus was not active and did not affect my lifestyle in any significant way.

It was eight months after delivering Seth when my lupus flared with a vengeance. It attacked all my major joints and connective tissues. I moved around with a pair of crutches, pureed my food and sucked it through a thin straw because it was impossible to move my inflamed jaw. I was finally officially diagnosed with lupus after four months of a desperate search for a cure. The rheumatologist also discovered that I had an anti-Roh antigen which may have caused clotting of the blood when my lupus became active during my late pregnancy. This was most likely the reason for Seth's unstable growth.

At two-and-a-half years of age, Seth was diagnosed with autism spectrum disorder. It was a shattering moment for us. It took us nearly two years of waiting before he was finally enrolled into one of the two special schools providing subsidized intervention programs for children with autism. In Singapore special education does not come under the purview of the Ministry of Education but is left to charity organisations to manage. In the meantime, out of desperation, as early treatment in autism is crucial, we turned to the privately run centres and paid exorbitant prices to receive basic support for speech, behaviour, occupational and bio-medical therapies. Seth had brought us on our first roller-coaster ride and we were afraid.

It took us three years to embrace that fear and to try for another child. Still today, the actual cause of autism is much disputed among researchers and doctors. While some believe it could be caused by prenatal or postnatal trauma, others believe strongly that it is due to an immunity breakdown because of vaccine toxicity. Yet others claim that it is hereditary, since it occurs more often in boys than in girls, although a gene responsible for this has yet to be identified. The questions 'What if?' and 'Are you sure you want to take the risk?' kept popping out from the mouths of our concerned family and friends. Some thought our decision was plain foolishness as my lupus has been shown to be more active during pregnancy. But we were certain that fear should not stop us from giving Seth a sibling to grow up with and to love.

It was another difficult pregnancy. I bled for six months, and had hormonal injections daily for three months to prevent miscarriage.

To control my lupus, I was prescribed a daily Clexane injection to dilute my blood, along with aspirin, oral steroid and medications for my hypothyroidism. On 22 December 2001, I delivered my second son, Jude, via caesarean section at 38 weeks as his growth rate had dropped significantly after the thirty-fifth week.

I quit my job as a manager with the Singapore Red Cross in June 2004 to focus on Seth's growing needs. I had all my plans beautifully laid out – I was a good strategist. Exactly two months later, I discovered that I was pregnant yet again. I was in shock. We were already surviving on a single income and struggling with Seth's expensive intervention programs and now this! How was I going to go through another nine months of expensive and painful treatment, not to mention the deep daily anxiety? How were we going to cope? But Seth had taught us well. We took a deep breath and once again said 'Yes' to life. We were ready to take another roller-coaster ride.

It proved to be the hardest of my three pregnancies. I had constant nausea and was exhausted every moment of the day. All my medications were again increased to prevent a possible flare of lupus. I remembered 27 August 2004 so well. It was the day my nausea lifted and I started to glow, or so everyone said. It was also the day I went for a thorough scan at thirteen weeks at the hospital, as I had refused the standard amniocentesis test strongly recommended by most gynaecologists for women above 35 years in Singapore. I was 40 years of age and I was told that it was a routine procedure.

I was not anxious as I had been taking the same precautions I took for my second successful pregnancy. Midway through the scan, the chatty radiographer went silent and wouldn't look at me. My heart skipped a few beats and started racing madly. It's just your imagination, I consoled myself. Two doctors rushed into the room and started talking to each other in muted undertones.

Then one of the doctors looked at me and announced quietly, 'We detected something that shouldn't be there.' When I probed for more details, he added, 'The results will be out in two hours time; I suggest that you bring the results back to your gynaecologist and discuss the options with him.' Options! A nice word used to mean a situation bad enough to consider abortion. I had never felt so alone in all my life. I told myself to be brave, called Jega on my mobile and sobbed my heart out in the anonymity of a female toilet.

Our little baby had cystic hygroma, a condition where there is a collection of brain and spinal fluid around the neck of the fetus. Our baby also displayed thick folds around the neck region, which was consistent with Down or Turner's syndrome. We were told that her condition was so severe that death inside my womb or a few days after delivery was a certainty. We were advised to prepare for the worst as the massive volume of fluid, which measured 8 mm x 12.3 mm in circumference on her 3.7 cm long body, would likely choke the baby in a few months time as it made its way to the lungs.

In the three weeks before our next appointment, I mourned bitterly for the loss of a normal pregnancy and I prepared for the death of my child. I called my rheumatologist to check if I should stop my expensive daily injections as there was no hope of survival for the baby anyway. It was then that I was informed that the diagnosis had also indicated that there was a tiny chance of survival for the baby but it would be born with severe disabilities. It was a heart-breaking moment of truth for me and I panicked.

The future was so bleak and dark and each time I ventured there, my heart shrank and wilted in my chest. I thought of the many severely disabled children I had met in Seth's special school arriving in their parent's arms, helpless as newborns. How often had I looked on with compassion, secretly thankful that this time it was not me. How seductive then was the thought of ending all this pain and uncertainty. A second disabled child – please, no! I understood why abortion often seemed to be the perfect answer; it was so practical on a certain plane, and it 'solves' everything. Life could go back to normal again. Ahh, that word again – *normal* – such a balm to the senses. I could focus on Seth's needs and help Jude to grow up well – just the way Jega and I had planned it all when I gave up my job.

But my little one had a chance to live on, and deep in my heart I knew that he or she had a right to live. How could I deny the scans I had been seeing at the gynaecologist's clinic – the bravely beating heart, a fully formed brain and all those undeniably human fingers and toes? Jega and I decided that we wanted this baby, that we were meant to have three unique children.

Most of our family members and friends were very supportive of our decision; others expressed shock that we could even contemplate keeping the baby. 'How could you bear to bring a child to suffer like that? It is better for all to just terminate the pregnancy! Think of your suffering and the immense medical cost you're going to bear for the rest of your life,' they advised in all sincerity. I held back the truth from many whom I knew would react negatively to our situation. I lost my confidence in carrying on bravely with the pregnancy, especially in the presence of medical professionals. My rheumatologist advised me to stop my injections because the 'medical diagnosis points to the fact there is no point in sustaining the pregnancy at this level.' The nurse assisting me to the examination table at the maternity clinic shook her head sympathetically and pronounced with a heavy sigh: 'I've seen many cases like this; they have no chance of survival. Your fetus looks so bad, better not to let it live – you can always try again.' Our paediatrician confirmed that medical literature has shown that in rare cases the hygroma may resolve itself but such babies would usually 'be left with Turner's syndrome and would be intellectually slow.'

I walked the tight-rope between hope and fear almost every day for the next six months. How far were we going to go to stop suffering from walking into our lives when it was so much a part of being human? We told the baby we wanted her – in whatever package she was coming in. And she would be beautiful to us. We willed her to live on every day, every moment. I deliberately put on my make-up with care every day. I dressed up. Jega and I started dating each other every Friday either for a movie, our favourite Japanese meal or a simple cup of tea at rustic Serangoon Road. We were determined to celebrate the life in me.

On 17 September our gynaecologist, staring intently at the scan monitor, gave a start of surprise. In a very careful tone he commented that the hygroma appeared to be shrinking. Hope stirred in our hearts. Three weeks later he couldn't find the hygroma on the screen at all. On 29 October I went for a repeat thorough scan at the same hospital on the advice of the gynae-cologist. It was a different radiographer. Like the previous lady, she started out friendly and chatty and asked me if it was my first visit to the hospital. It was obvious to me then that by some strange stroke of luck she had not checked on my previous records and did not know of the earlier diagnosis. I did not enlighten her as I wanted to receive a totally unbiased diagnosis.

Then, for what seemed like ages, she kept working silently. Déjà vu. Then she coyly asked if we wanted a boy or a girl. It was the last thing on our minds! I held my breath – can this be true? Can miracles really happen to us? Let it happen, please! The doctor walked in, sat down and scanned each picture in silence. Then he asked pleasantly if my husband would like to come in for the results. Everyone was relaxed; I was desperate to know what they were seeing. Everything seemed to stand still.

'Congratulations! You have a healthy baby girl.'

Jega and I rushed back to the clinic with the results, hearts bursting with happiness. My gynaecologist was beaming, sharing our contagious joy. 'I don't know what to say, I've never seen anything like this in my thirty years of practice!' Those who did not support our decision gasped in disbelief at the news and congratulated us with some degree of awkwardness. Our families and friends shouted with joy and believed once again in the impossible. Jega and I went to the park, sat on a bench and cried and laughed in each other's arms.

We finally met Sonia Grace, our teacher of hearts, on a lovely Friday morning in mid-February 2005. She was pronounced perfectly healthy, with no trace of any disability or abnormality after a series of chromosomal tests ordered by the paediatrician. As I hold her, I see the excess loose skin around the back of her neck, the only reminder to us of her heroic struggle with the fatal hygroma. She smiles in her sleep and reminds us that life is an adventure, a ride we have to learn to embrace without looking back too often in regret or too far ahead in fear.

Today at seven years of age, Seth continues to struggle with his autism; he shuts his ears to the sound of the whistling wind and stares at our window grills for hours. He has yet to call me Mum. Jude is a healthy, talkative little joy who shows me what Seth will be like one day. I thank Sonia for teaching me that the most beautiful ceiling in the world is a perfectly blue sky with puffy white clouds floating on it and that the sweetest music ever heard is the gurgling first laughter of a 3-month-old child.

There is really no such thing as an ordinary life because we are all – every little one of us, born and unborn – extraordinary individuals, uniquely crafted, for a purpose we can only find out if we dare to live without too much fear.

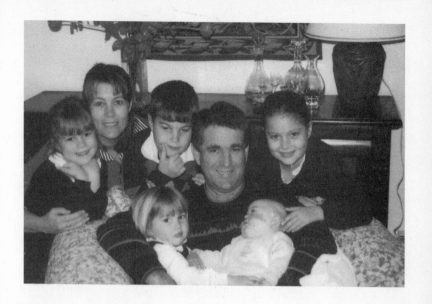

Julia Anderson

Julia Anderson lives on a 4000-acre wheat and cattle property in Gunnedah, NSW, with her four children and her husband, who was the Deputy Prime Minister of Australia until he stepped down for family reasons in June 2005. She is enjoying her new position as chief cattle musterer on the property.

Julia Anderson

FINDING JOY IN THE WEAK AMONG US

Picture this: My 7-year-old son has risen at daylight. Quietly he moves to the cot of his 3-month-old brother Andrew. Andrew stops crying as he is gently rolled over. Nick delicately places him in his bouncer. Carefully, but with clear purpose, he harnesses Andrew and his bouncer to himself. Once in harness the sleigh is ready to fly. My darling eldest boy begins galloping down the hall. He is a sturdy and willing reindeer and Andrew is Santa Claus.

I step into the hallway to find out what is happening. There I see a gleeful big boy playing with his long-awaited brother. Andrew, his baby cheeks made round by an open-mouthed grin, is cooing with pure excitement. And his big brother is feeling the thrill of finally being able to play with him. I smile and tears well and fall amidst a turmoil of joy and fear.

* * *

It slowly dawned on me over a few weeks that perhaps I was pregnant. I was 35. We already had four children – three daughters and a son. I felt surprised and excited. One Sunday on the way home from church we stopped at the chemist to pick up a pregnancy testing kit. Soon I knew we had another child on the way. I broke the scary but exciting news to my husband.

Being a naturally optimistic person, my first thoughts were of the joy and increased pleasure this new member would bring to our family. It is not like me to focus on the negatives. My glass is always half full, never half empty. This new child was neither planned nor unwelcomed. This was an undeniable blessing in my book. I felt a huge overwhelming happiness – even if a little daunted at the prospect of the additional workload with an often-absent husband.

Wouldn't it be good to have another boy, I thought. Then everyone would have a brother and sisters. As time went on I felt my baby move. This fuelled my excitement. And though I had never wanted to know the sex of a baby before, I was keen to find out this time. When I went along to my first routine ultrasound, the technician asked if I wanted to know whether I was carrying a boy or a girl. I couldn't resist. She said, 'This baby is a boy.' I felt tears of joy trickle down my cheeks – the first of many tears I was to shed for our little son Andrew.

The technician kept going with her measurements and checks. I was floating on the good news of another boy for the family. She mentioned that she couldn't find his stomach, but not to worry. 'Just come back tomorrow when the baby has had a drink and perhaps we will be able to see his stomach then.'

The next day I went back for another ultrasound. The doctor and the technician were there. I was still floating and happy. The doctor was straight-talking and calm. 'This baby's stomach is not showing up. It will be there, but it has no fluid in it. The most likely cause is an oesophageal defect.'

My mind was crowded with questions. What is that? What does this mean? What can be done about it? Help! I don't know what this is about. All his other measurements were very positive.

The next stop was a paediatric surgeon. In a few weeks I was sitting in his office. He reassured me this problem was entirely fixable. The baby would need surgery soon after birth because his oesophagus was not joined onto his stomach. This was an operation he had performed before and he felt quite confident about the outcome. I felt soothed and comforted by this news. It could be fixed. He would be able to carry on like a normal child within a few weeks or months of the operation.

More ultrasounds were recommended as I was likely to retain significant amounts of fluid as Andrew wasn't swallowing and processing the amniotic fluid. I needed close monitoring. All seemed to go well for the next few ultrasounds. The doctor then suggested I have a few more tests so he could deal effectively with our son when he was born. So I kept my positive outlook and waited for the test results.

Several days later, on a fresh winter morning, I was at home with my two youngest girls, two plumbers and two tilers. The two older children were at school. The house was alive with noise and dust and workmen's chatter. If we were to have five children sharing a bathroom, it would need a robust re-fit.

The phone rang. I went to my bedroom to answer it. It was my obstetrician. What I heard was not what I was expecting. Our baby had Down syndrome. This news absolutely took my breath away. I remember the long involuntary gasp that passed through my throat. The doctor was talking and I was in a numb, sad, almost void place. I sat down involuntarily onto the bed with a thump, holding my tummy with tears rolling down my cheeks.

I suddenly wanted more than anything to be alone. No plumbers, no tilers, no questions about tile and tap placements. I wanted the comfort and peace of my home restored. I had to ring John.

My husband was in the middle of a speech to firemen when I rang him on his mobile phone. He was congratulating them on their sterling efforts in fighting the fires in the Pilliga Scrub months before. Though I wanted to talk to him, I was surprised when he answered. He said, 'Darling, I am in the middle of my speech; what is it?' I said, 'This news is more important than whatever you are doing now – you have to know this, our baby has

Down syndrome.'

John coped amazingly well. Together we were shattered. Already we were anticipating what was ahead for Baby Andrew – the possible operations, the uncertainties, the pain – as well as the fear and sadness the other children would feel. Yet, serving as a Cabinet Minister, in public, John kept his head up and focused on his job.

It was hard for him and it was hard for us. We had four gorgeous children already. What had happened to this little man in my womb? What would he need from us? We loved him already. We wanted to defend him and make sure he was healed and happy, but would this be possible?

The remaining weeks of my pregnancy were full of ultrasounds, tests, and doctors' visits. The doctors who cared for Andrew and me were fantastic all along the way. They answered all our questions and helped us to understand Down syndrome as much as they were able.

Since there is a huge range of possible complications associated with Down syndrome, there was much about Andrew we could not know before he was born. It was like waiting for a package to be delivered: we knew a parcel was coming – we just didn't know what would be in it.

For us there was never any question of abortion. It may sound strange, but I didn't even think of it because to me he was already our son. I had already felt him moving inside me for months. He was our child – as deserving of our love and protection as any of our other children. Abortion was just not an option we thought of for Andrew. Sadly, we learned from our doctor that of four Down syndrome babies diagnosed in utero the same month as Andrew, we were the only couple proceeding with the pregnancy.

I thought often of my childhood. For a while our family had taken care of a child with a disability. One thing I came to know

was how cruel other people and children could be toward someone who appeared different. I remembered the stares, those
penetrating unfriendly stares of people which revealed their fear
and doubts and questions. How could we bear those stares and
cruel taunts for one of our own children? How could we protect
a child from that? I was also aware of the extra care and time a
child with physical complications would need.

The fact of already having four healthy, bouncy children, made
the last weeks of the pregnancy both good and bad. It was great
to appreciate afresh just how blessed we were to have such terrific,
resilient children. The routines of caring for them – the continuing
of birthday parties, swimming lessons, homework, taking the dog
for a walk – all the things which link together the days of normal
family life, were a welcomed distraction from worrying about
what might lie ahead.

On the down side, of course, was my declining energy level.
Mothering four children requires energy and imagination. As
Andrew grew and his birth day came closer, the combination of
anticipating an unknown future and carrying a growing baby
made me feel tired in every possible way. As an added complication, I was blowing up like a balloon with the extra fluid Andrew
was not drinking. A couple of times I had to have fluid – up to a
litre at a time – removed through a needle inserted into my
stomach. Happily, John scooped up the children in early January
and took them away on holidays, while I stayed behind to stay
close to the hospital and the doctors.

A friend came to stay during that time and we did lots of
tidying, nesting, and re-arranging jobs which are difficult to do
with a house full of family. I rested and enjoyed the sprucing-up
of the home. As it turned out, the timing of that little interlude
was perfect. The children and John were refreshed, the house was
improved and I was rested. It was all just in time for Andrew's

premature arrival on the very day his brother turned seven – 31 January 1998.

Although Andrew was six weeks early, the birth itself was reasonably straightforward. He was beautiful – much more 'normal-looking' than I had expected. However, the usual cuddling, relief and joy which occurs moments after the birth of a child never happened with Andrew. Because of his oesophageal defect, he could not be cuddled for long, or fed at my breast like the others. This was the first moment where the anticipation of pain became a reality. My beautiful Andrew was taken away for testing and assistance pretty much straight away after he was born. He returned intubated – a tube in his nose to suction saliva, and a 'button' in his tummy where he would be fed.

It was very difficult not to feel that Andrew, John and I had been cheated of a very special and important moment, but this was how it had to be for Andrew if he were to survive and thrive. It was not just me and the family that he needed for his happiness and contentment. It was much, much more than we as a family were able to provide. Andrew needed doctors and nurses and specialised equipment and monitoring and testing. He needed miracles.

I retired from the delivery suite to a private room without a baby. I felt sad and tense. I was an experienced mother, and yet there was so little I could do for him. I expressed milk which he received through a tube, changed his nappy, stroked him, prayed, and watched as others cared for him. At night, in hospital, I slept while Andrew was tended in the intensive care nursery. This was a very different pattern of care and I felt at times almost out of the loop.

This separation grew more intense when I was discharged from hospital after the birth. Going home without a baby was a strain. And it seemed that every day brought more news of hurdles for

Andrew.

His tiny heart would need surgery, but only after his throat and oesophageus were repaired. Then there were bowel problems (Hirschsprung's) which required immediate surgery and then follow-up surgery somewhere down the track. Each time I went to hospital there were more briefings from doctors and nurses.

Externally Andrew was gorgeous, but inside the story was so different. The basic message from our very caring neonatologist was this: as far as internal complications for Down syndrome went, Andrew had just about all of them. This was an enormous blow. We had researched the condition before Andrew's birth and we knew there was much to be hopeful about. Many people with Down syndrome live quite normally, function well as adults and make a great contribution to their families and communities. But our dear Andrew had a body which was working against him, not for him.

It took time to prepare for the oesophagus repair surgery. The doctors knew from X-rays that the distance between the ending of Andrew's oesophagus and the tube on his stomach was greater than had ever been successfully rejoined before. After much consultation, they decided to attempt the repair. At first the surgeon was hopeful, but the reality which followed was heart-wrenching. The operation was a success, but we quickly found that the site of the join kept growing closed. The doctors had done everything in their power. It was grim for them too. They wanted to be able to help Andrew.

One night he started to swell, and the stitches across his back popped open. We were called in to the hospital in the wee small hours, as one of his lungs had collapsed. He was frighteningly close to death, and yet stoically pulled through. Many operations followed to force his throat open. Each time Andrew was operated on he would fight to recover. He often contracted post-operative pneumonia. Occasionally the 'button' in his tummy, through which he was fed by tube, would fall out. When this occurred the acid from his stomach would leak out onto his skin and cause him terrible pain.

I can't remember now exactly how many times Andrew went to surgery, but I remember that his surgeries often went over time. The time for the end of the surgery would come and go, and we would still be in the waiting room, waiting for news of Andrew.

I well remember the joy of seeing Andrew without any new tubes for the first time. A few days later we were able to take him home. Amazing support was available for Andrew's care at home. We were visited by a speech pathologist and a physiotherapist, but it was pretty scary looking after him. He still had his colostomy bag, and was fed through his stomach 'button'. It wasn't long before he was back in hospital for his next throat opening operation.

After several subsequent attempts to repair Andrew's oesophagus, he fell gravely ill with pneumonia. Andrew had been home with us for less than three weeks in the first five months of his life.

I cannot fault any of the medical team who cared for Andrew and our family. They were considerate of us as a family and treated all of us with equal love and respect. They reached out to each of the children and made them feel involved and informed.

It was one of the nursing staff who gently took me aside one day to talk with me about the ever-increasing possibility that Andrew might not survive. She was gentle and caring. She wanted to know whether I might like to take him home to care for him with palliative care support. His pneumonia was severe. She could see that the unnatural divide between home and hospital was taking its toll. She was also willing to be honest with me about what her years of experience had taught her: we needed to start preparing ourselves for the possibility of his death.

So we took our dear boy home and set up a de facto hospital room in the dining room. A palliative care nurse visited, usually twice a day. Oxygen was delivered to our house and I had a veritable army of carers: family, church friends, neighbours and so many other wonderful people who all pitched in to help us care for Andrew at home. Our older children needed to keep their lives going and Andrew needed constant care.

Andrew smiled at us when his pain relief medication was at work. He wanted to live and enjoy us. He loved his siblings and he loved his parents. He suffered immensely. He snatched moments in between sickness and pain to be happy and joyous. To see such a tiny boy with so much to cope with flash a smile was worth all the struggle and heartache.

Our eldest daughter came to me one day in tears. A child with Down syndrome had been in her year three class. She had not reached out to her as fully as she should have. Now, after knowing Andrew, she felt guilty and sad for not having tried to make a friendship with one of her peers who was different.

Through his pain and the turmoil of his short and difficult life, Andrew was overhauling our family on the inside. He was at work changing our souls in a way that only he could. He was teaching us that external appearances, physical disabilities and even grotesque pain were not the most important things in life. From him we learned to look at our own imperfections differently. We learned to see that we are all imperfect, just in different ways.

Andrew's physical imperfections were killing him and yet, as we watched him snatch moments of happiness from the jaws of death, we were completely rearranged emotionally. He was the tiniest and most vulnerable of the lot of us, and from him we learned about real strength. What were any of our perceived struggles, compared to what he was going through? Did we cry out to God for healing for Andrew? Were we perplexed about why this happened? Did we wish things were different? Absolutely yes. Did we experience all sorts of varying advice and unhelpful comments from well-meaning people who didn't know what to say? Absolutely yes. Did some people comfort us in ways that still touches us today? Absolutely yes.

Family and close friends gathered at our home as Andrew lay dying. We had round-the-clock helpers. Andrew was nestled in someone's arms constantly. His oxygen, antibiotics and morphine were all at hand, and helpfully administered by palliative care nurses.

On 7 August 1998, Andrew's body completely failed him and he died surrounded by John, my mother and father, and me. Andrew died because his little body was overwhelmed with pneumonia and so many other compounding abnormalities. But before he left us, this small cheerful soul left behind a storehouse of memories and lessons which we are still mining today.

We had some very beautiful encouragements which nourished our battered hearts during our sojourn with Andrew. Below I have included the most helpful ones which may be a help to someone else in a similar circumstance.

Our minister asked me early on if I was enjoying my baby. Honestly, I wasn't. I was crying for him, praying for him, fearing for him and hoping the pain would stop, but I wasn't enjoying him. This one question changed my attitude to my hospital visits for the good. I started enjoying my little baby.

The following fable 'Welcome to Holland' was given to us when we first discovered Andrew had Down syndrome. It really helped me re-orientate myself to life with Andrew. And it was the beginning of understanding how to re-arrange my expectations.

'Welcome to Holland'
Emily Pearl Kingsley

I am often asked to describe the experience of raising a child with a disability – to try to help people who have not shared that unique experience to understand it, to imagine how it would feel. It's like this . . .

When you are going to have a baby, it's like planning a fabulous vacation trip to Italy. You buy a bunch of guidebooks and make your wonderful plans. The Colosseum. The Michaelangelo 'David'. The gondolas in Venice. You may learn some handy phrases in Italian. It's all very exciting. After months of eager anticipation, the day finally arrives. You pack your bags and off you go.

Several hours later, the plane lands. The stewardess comes in and says, 'Welcome to Holland.' 'Holland?' you say; 'What do you mean, Holland? I signed up for Italy! I'm supposed to be in Italy. All my life I've dreamed of going to Italy.' But there's been a change in flight plan. They've landed in Holland and there you must stay.

The important thing is that they haven't taken you to a horrible, disgusting, filthy place, full of pestilence, famine and disease. It's just a different place. So you must go out and buy more guidebooks. And you must learn a whole new language. And you will meet a whole new group of people you would never have met.

It's just a different place. It's slower-paced than Italy, less flashy than Italy. But after you've been there for a while and you catch your breath, you look around and you begin to notice that Holland has windmills, Holland has tulips, Holland even has Rembrandts.

But everyone you know is busy coming and going from Italy, and they're all bragging about what a wonderful time they had there. And for the rest of your life, you will say, 'Yes, that's where I was supposed to go. That's what I had planned.' And the pain of that will never, ever, ever go away, because the loss of that dream is a very significant loss. But if you spend your life mourning the fact that you didn't get to Italy, you may never be free to enjoy the very special, the very lovely things about Holland.

The last thing I have to share with you is the eulogy John gave at Andrew's funeral. It gave voice to much of the struggle we had been through since the very beginning of the news about Andrew until the day he left us. Perhaps these things can help others to recover from the shock of changed expectations and unexpected blessings from the suffering our world sometimes serves us.

Eulogy by John Anderson, Monday 10 August 1998,
St Matthew's Anglican Church, Wanniassa, Canberra

Andrew

Andrew's life saw us often wondering what we'd done to deserve so much difficulty.

His passing sees us wondering what we did to deserve so rich a blessing as his short six-month life was ultimately to be.

This little fellow was quite defenceless – more so by far than even an ordinary baby – yet he was to totally and utterly disarm us.

He was devoid of all earthly power – yet was to speak to us more powerfully than all the clever words that I could spin together as a Cabinet Minister.

He, quite helpless, needing everything done for him, revealed much to us about our own feelings, weaknesses and inadequacies.

Unable himself to choose between selfishness and selflessness he made me, at least, very conscious of my own selfishness – my desire to stay within my own 'comfort zone'.

We who have so much, take so much for granted, always seem to think we deserve and need more; how we are shown up by those who struggle simply to live.

And how ungrateful we must seem to God.

Andrew taught me, who, from time to time, railed against God for the burden I felt he was adding to an already burdened life, that I had a lot to learn about loving and accepting others without reservation.

For that is what God offers us even though we are nowhere near as attractive as we might like to think we are.

I started to realise these truths as I considered how, if God hates selfishness and vanity and greed, who really had the problem – Andrew? or me?

And what of the marks of character that he did reveal? His courage, his warmth, his tolerance in the face of awful suffering?

Certainly others saw, and I came to see more clearly, that the girl I married had all these qualities and more – Julia's love for that little boy, her strength, her resolve, and courage were inspirational.

Well, Andrew, we gave you what we could, but you gave us more. A team of dedicated and skilled medical people performed miracles, but it was not to be: you knew more pain and suffering in your six months than most of us experience in our lifetimes, so while we thank God for you, we thank God, too, for taking you home.

You go with our love and quiet confidence that you form the advance party for your Mum and Dad, and Jessica, Nick, Georgie and Laura.

We have learnt that God's response to our difficulties is not often so much to remove them, but rather to provide us with the strength to carry on.

Above all, you see, through you God taught us something we'd heard about but not really understood as well as we should.

That His grace is sufficient for us, for his power is made perfect in weakness – that is of course, the message of a broken Jesus on the cross.

God's grace was sufficient, is sufficient, will be sufficient.

There can be no greater blessing than knowing this truth.

Perhaps the most important thing to be gained from Andrew's life is that in the midst of shocking suffering, you can find joy and purpose in the tiniest and weakest amongst us. And from their brave hearts we learn a bit more about how to live, order our priorities, and value what is really important in life.

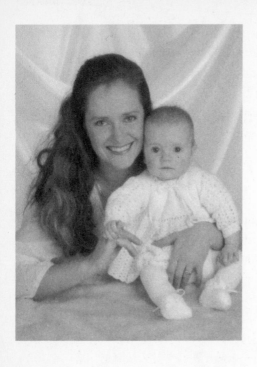

Karalyn McDonald

Karalyn McDonald is a PhD researcher who held a National Health and Medical Research Council (NHMRC) scholarship for her current project, HIV-positive women, pregnancy and motherhood. She has published in professional journals on the gender differences between HIV-positive women and men in relation to antiretroviral uptake as well as the identities HIV-positive people assign themselves, and the role of motherhood in the lives of HIV-positive women in Australia. She has also presented at major HIV/AIDS conferences both nationally and internationally and is the principal author of the first monograph written about Australian HIV-positive women. Aside from her work, Karalyn's passions are her 2-year-old daughter and horse riding. A rider for twenty-five years, she has taken part in cross-country and showjumping events, concentrating on dressage for the last four years.

Karalyn McDonald

'THE BEST EXPERIENCE OF MY LIFE': HIV-POSITIVE WOMEN ON PREGNANCY AND BIRTH IN AUSTRALIA

Today more than 40 million people are estimated to be infected with HIV/AIDS and women make up around half of that figure. However in Australia, women make up only 7 percent of the total population of people living with HIV/AIDS. Due to Australia's vast geography and relatively small population, the 1320 women living with HIV are widely dispersed and many are therefore isolated and often not visible within the epidemic in Australia. The first woman was diagnosed with HIV in Australia in 1984. As of September 2004, 1598 have been diagnosed with HIV and 278 women have died from AIDS-related illnesses. Around three quarters of women are infected within heterosexual relationships (NCHECR, 2005).

Initially in western industrialised countries it was gay men who were hardest hit by this virus and women were considered involved only insofar as they were caregivers or mothers, sisters or friends of the gay men affected by HIV/AIDS. As the first few women were diagnosed they were categorised as either 'innocent victims' infected by 'bad blood' – a haemophiliac husband or medical malpractice – or were somehow 'deserving' by engaging in deviant behaviour such as sex work, substance abuse or promiscuous behaviour (Lawless et al., 1996). It became apparent early in the epidemic that this virus could also be passed from an HIV-infected mother to her baby and so lead to a new identity for

HIV-positive women who chose to continue with their pregnancies as 'vectors of disease' (Anastos & Marte, 1989; de Bruyn, 1998; Gorna, 1996).

Medical advances have reduced the risk of vertical transmission of HIV from mother to baby, yet HIV-positive women's desires to become mothers still meet with opposition because it clashes with what society deems to be a suitable or 'good mother'. Despite the passing of the twentieth anniversary of the discovery of HIV/AIDS, there is still considerable stigma and ignorance surrounding this virus. Due to this stigma experienced by many HIV-positive women today and the concerns they often have about confidentiality for their family and their children, the following chapter is based on excerpts from a number of women's stories rather than one woman's experience. All names and identifying details have been changed.

In the first decade of the epidemic, prognosis was dire and most people diagnosed with HIV were told they would live for between five and ten years. For those women who were already mothers the only course of action was to get their affairs in order, which of course included organising the future care of their children. However, for those women who had not yet had children, a diagnosis of HIV also appeared to be a diagnosis of childlessness.

Yvette, 39 and HIV-positive for fifteen years at the time of interview, was diagnosed early in the epidemic and did not have any children.

> I was diagnosed in '86. It was probably the motherhood thing that was the biggest impact for me than actually being told, 'You have got AIDS.' They were the words used, but I didn't have AIDS, I had HIV. But the language used back then was different. I was told I had a year to live and I couldn't have children. I came from being a drug user and a sex worker at that time and so I didn't have any self-esteem anyway, so the fact that I was going to die was no big

deal. But being told I couldn't have children *was* a big deal because I had a termination a couple of years previously. So it was not like being told you can't have children because your body is unable to, it's about having that choice taken away from you. The medical profession back then, it was like [they were giving me] an order, it wasn't like a choice or anything you had a say in. You were made to feel very guilty if you even contemplated the thought, and [you were] told that you could definitely give it to your child. So I would say for about the first two years after I was diagnosed, the time that I was crying was actually over the fact of not having children and having that taken away from me.

Layla, aged 33 and diagnosed ten years prior to interview, was advised against pregnancy:

I don't remember anyone telling me when I was diagnosed that I couldn't have children. But I remember a little while later talking through my prognosis and at that point in time they weren't looking past five years, and when I did broach the subject of children I was told that for a start it couldn't be guaranteed that I would be around to raise a child. The main thing that stuck with me was that there was no way of knowing what the impact of a pregnancy would have on my health, and the doctor said, 'We would advise against a pregnancy, not knowing those things'. So I basically just went along with that. I was really devastated. The more I thought about it, the more devastated I became. I realised that it was something that had been taken away from me . . . [because] I'd always thought about having kids; even when I was at school I always babysat.

Before treatments, the risk of vertical transmission of HIV from mother to baby was estimated to be between 25 and 30 percent, however, as can be seen from Yvette's story, most doctors deemed this risk to be unacceptable when combined with the uncertainty of the mother's prognosis. Yet not all women accepted this assessment and some women, like Sophie, did continue with their pregnancies despite medical advice to the contrary. Sophie was 39 and diagnosed ten years prior to interview:

Well, at first I thought I was sick; I didn't realise I was pregnant. But I was sick and I went to one of the local GPs [general practitioners]. There are clinics everywhere in this area, and I said, 'Look, I'm sick all the time. I'm never sick; what's wrong with me?' He said to me, 'I'll have to do some blood tests; I want to do blood tests. Can I test you for everything? Hepatitis, HIV and . . .' No, he didn't say HIV, he said AIDS, let's get that correct. He said AIDS. And I just said, 'Yeah, go for it; that's not going to happen to me,' because that wasn't a concern of mine. I had never been overly promiscuous. I had never shot up drugs or . . .

I came back on the Saturday morning to be told that I was HIV-positive and the reason I'm sick is because I'm pregnant, but don't worry about that because he's already arranged for me to have a termination . . . The doctor said to me that he couldn't really do anything for me. He didn't know. He had no proper training for HIV or anything like that, and that I should go to a different clinic that specialised in HIV. So I went to this clinic and they told me that there was no way I can have children. So I went and spoke to a girlfriend of mine that's HIV, and she actually told me to go to a particular hospital, because there was a female counsellor there. I found the counsellor very, very good, at the hospital, and she actually referred me to PAU (Paediatric AIDS Unit) at the Children's Hospital, and I went there and that was the biggest eye-opener, because their theory was, no, I didn't have to have a termination. I found the staff there were just awesome, and they were really, really good. We went through all the pros and the cons and how I had only recently acquired it and how my T-cells were better than the average person's, and my health was just A-1, and they said my chances of having a positive child would be one in twenty-seven or something around that. So we ummed and we ahhed, and I'm, like, oh, God! I'd booked for the termination but I couldn't go through with it; I got up and I left. Then she was born and because I was so uneducated they used her as a guinea pig. They pushed her, they poked her, they jabbed her. Luckily she was negative.

Sophie's experience of being advised to terminate her pregnancy was certainly not unique. Early in the epidemic many health care professionals advised terminations for pregnant HIV-positive women. Denise, 43 and diagnosed fifteen years prior to the interview, was the mother of one child when she received her diagnosis.

I first found out about being HIV-positive and being pregnant at the same time. That was a real surprise. I didn't expect to be either. I didn't even think about it. It was just a subconscious thing. I said to the doctor I actually thought it was my hepatitis [C] playing up. So when I got those results, my son was about five or six years old at the time, and for me being pregnant was the bigger issue. Like, the HIV was, 'Oh, wow'. But the hardest thing was the decision about the pregnancy. They said, 'Well, you've got to have a termination.' Now I say that I made that decision but I was greatly influenced. I regret what I did then but they said to me, 'You've got a 6-year-old son; who's going to look after him? You're going to get sick; your baby may be sick.' And I remember asking them – standing in the corridor there – and I remember saying, 'Isn't there another woman in the whole of Australia who's ever been in my situation?' And they said, 'Oh, not that we know of.' But they gave me an A4 sheet about women in Africa, and I can just remember thinking to myself I couldn't connect that situation with my situation, and I had, like, zilch knowledge about HIV. And in fact now, knowing all that I do, we weren't even given it because I don't think it was available. It was like, 'Well, go home and die', basically. My partner and I sort of didn't talk about all this hard stuff, but reluctantly I had a termination and unfortunately that wasn't successful the first time. I didn't realise, and went back because I was haemorrhaging and was really crook, and they said a bit of the foetus was left behind. So I sort of had, like, two, but it was really one. It was a really traumatic experience and I remember crying heaps.

Yet even with the advent of treatments and the subsequent reduction in the risk of vertical transmission of HIV from mother to baby, some HIV-positive women were still advised by their health care professionals to have a termination. Brooke was diagnosed in 1994 and fell pregnant in 1996:

I went in to a doctor's appointment to speak to someone and I was supposed to go in to have a blood test because I had heard about this viral load test that was really new then. And I thought, oh, maybe I should have a blood test and find out what my viral load is, and my T-cell count, and that will determine whether I will have the child or not. I went to the doctor and I just didn't like the feeling of the doctor, and she was saying, 'Come back tomorrow for a blood test,' and I was thinking, 'I'm not coming back here.' She was saying that the viral load was not that important, which now they know that it really is. And maybe she could sense that I was a bit confused about the whole thing, and she was being a bit pessimistic, saying, 'Let's face it, maybe you're not going to be here; maybe you'll die.' That sort of thing. It just felt like she was scaring me into not going through with it [the birth]. So then I had an abortion.

Lily, 35, found out she was pregnant the year after she was diagnosed HIV-positive, six years before the interview:

Then I got pregnant in 1996 with Zach. I didn't find out I was pregnant until I was four months. So I booked an abortion; the doctors were virtually begging me to get rid of it. They made my decision to abort. But then I saw Zach on the screen when they did the ultrasound, and once I saw his eyes, he spoke to me: 'How dare you . . .' were the words he was saying to me because the abortion was booked. The doctors and nurses were saying, 'Don't have the baby,' and forcing drugs onto me . . . They went along with me making the decision because I just couldn't do it, couldn't abort it. I couldn't believe I was pregnant – I had had two periods so I went to three doctors to verify that I was pregnant. I didn't have a stomach, nothing. It was a gift from God because I remember conception too. I asked for a baby so he is definitely a gift.

Early in the epidemic, medical opposition to HIV-positive women becoming mothers actually led to some women being sterilised. Laura and Audrey both underwent sterilisation and both felt they were given little choice but to comply with the medical advice. Laura, 39, was diagnosed along with her husband, eleven years before the interview:

Within a month of diagnosis I was sent to a gynaecologist. I saw him on a Tuesday and I had to fast on the Thursday night and on Friday I had 'elective' surgery at a major hospital and they sterilised me. I don't remember any of the process in terms of being able to recollect it. I am sure that I signed the consent form and I argued with them bitterly because Stuart had to sign the consent form, and I thought, 'This is *my* body; what has it got to do *him*?' You know, that whole feminist thing of 'Why is *he* having to sign?' Because it had nothing to do with him, and that's the only thing I remember about it, is being really indignant that my husband had to sign the consent form. I have no recollection about the counselling that they gave me apart from some really patronising nurse telling me that I was doing the right thing. I remember that because it was the pat on the back; you know, 'You're doing the right thing, love,' and they did that within a month [of diagnosis]. I think I just mentioned that we weren't quite sure what to do about contraception, and that was it; gone.

At the time the idea of having more children . . . I actually thought I was really lucky because I had a child who was negative, who was my husband's child, so I would have something of him when he did die, and she looks so much like her father that it does help in that continuation stuff. It's true that immortality comes through your children.

Laura's husband Stuart died within two years of their diagnosis, but Laura stayed well and went on to re-partner:

. . . [T]he idea of not actually having another baby, sometimes it hurts, though. Like after seeing my partner with his daughter and I think what it would be like. That whole female thing that we have about [how] it would be 'our child', and that is really difficult at times, and I have never had a chance to grieve for the fact that I couldn't have any more children; there was no time for that. I was too busy grieving for my husband, for all of the other stuff. One of the really awful things about diagnosis is that they don't give you time to grieve for the losses that aren't necessarily real, but those perceived losses are just as real for you, and you don't get that chance to grieve. I have never had a chance to grieve for the loss of the children that I probably never would have had. But that choice was taken away from me, and I never ever had a chance to grieve for that loss of choice. It still rears its ugly head when I go to the retreats and the women are there. There are always pregnant women on these bloody retreats, and I look at them and they are always glowing and wonderful and all that, and I think, yeah, it still hurts. There is a little ache that no matter how much therapy

I have been through, no matter how many times we have talked about it, yeah, it's still there.

Audrey, a mother of four, was also sterilised shortly after she was diagnosed in 1993. At 45, and eight years after diagnosis, she still finds her sterilisation painful to recall:

> When I was diagnosed and finally met up with my doctor – which would have been about six months later – the first thing I was told was, 'We would like to sterilise you.' They were the words he used and it really hit me, and it hurt, because I thought, well, they're not giving you a choice, they are kind of giving you a command. Because it was a decision my [second] husband and I made not to have children, so at that time I thought, okay, I'll go ahead with that. But it still hurt. It was about a year later my husband said that he would like to have a child and by that time I said, 'Well, it's too late. The decision has been made.' But I did think it would have been nice to give him a child.

Medical professionals were not the only people opposing HIV-positive women becoming mothers. Some women like Miranda and Layla experienced opposition from family and friends as well. Miranda, 36, was diagnosed ten years before the interview.

> With both pregnancies, I've said [they] were accidents, because it's really hard. People accept it better if you say, 'Oh, I accidentally fell pregnant and now I'm going through with it,' rather than saying, 'Oh this is my situation and I want a child,' because they consider that selfish. That was the problem with the termination that I had [the first time I was pregnant]. [When I told people] I had such negative reactions from people, saying, 'How could you? You won't be around to bring the child up. What if the child's sick?' And all the rest of it, and these were from friends. And if I had not told anyone, it would have been different, but because I

was on my own, I wasn't strong enough to . . . and because I didn't know anyone else. I had phone contact with positive women, but no one that I knew, really knew. If I had been in the situation I am in now then it would've been different.

Miranda and her husband both wanted to have children and Miranda soon fell pregnant again. This time, with the support of her husband, she gave birth to their son, Nathan. Miranda went on to have a second son five years later.

When I was pregnant with Jack, people – even family – were a bit, like, 'Oh, how could you do it again? You should just be happy that you have one child that is well. How could you go through the whole thing again?' It is like they think it is a bit greedy. So, again, I said it was an accident. There is this sense of shame. I felt guilty and ashamed when I was pregnant, like I couldn't really enjoy it because pregnancy is supposed to be this real spiritual thing, but I felt embarrassed when I was pregnant. Especially when, in between having Nathan and Jack, I was working in childcare and I got outed there by someone and I lost my job over it. He didn't fire me, but I'd been working 24 hours a week and then the next day, after he called me in the office, he said, 'Oh, someone said this about you; is it true?' And I said, 'Well, yes it is.' I think he expected me to quit, so my hours went from 24 hours a week to 8 hours a week. I stuck it out for six months but it was such hard going, and in the end I gave up after six months. So there was a feeling when I was pregnant with Jack, I didn't know who knew about my [HIV] status, so I'd be in the shopping mall and I'd be really paranoid because I found out who it was that had revealed it. It was someone who had heard it through gossip, so it was just a feeling of paranoia the whole time. So that was pretty yucky.

Layla also experienced a lack of support from friends and family:

It is funny, when I told friends I was pregnant some of them reacted very strangely, and later when I discussed it with them, they said, 'Well, we didn't know whether you were happy about it or not.' So I had to say to people, 'I am pregnant and I'm really happy about it,' so that they could react in the way they should. My family were really shocked about my decision and weren't very supportive. They were concerned that the impact on my health would be too great. I found out after I had the baby that they had had a family meeting about who would look after the baby when I died; [it] would have been nice to include me.

In 1994, the AIDS Clinical Trial Group (ACTG) 076 revealed that zidovudine (AZT) antepartum and then postpartum to the infant could radically alter the chance of vertical transmission of HIV from mother to baby from around 25 to 30 percent to approximately 8 percent. The implications of this study were to have an enormous effect on the lives of HIV-positive pregnant women, providing them with great hope and some sense of relief. The HIV/AIDS epidemic was further radically altered with the advent of new treatments, known as combination therapy, in 1996. These treatments significantly improved prospects for the clinical management of HIV and attendant diseases for many people living with HIV/AIDS and, in addition to other medical interventions, further reduced vertical transmission to less than 2 percent. Access to these treatments has generally been accepted by HIV-positive women as an effective way to reduce the risk of vertical transmission and potentially boost the health of the mother if needed, despite many women's concerns about the side effects of treatment and potential toxicity for both mother and baby.

Layla found her HIV specialist was supportive of her decision to get pregnant once they became aware of the ACTG 076 trials, however, the obstetrician she was referred to was less supportive:

I was put in touch with an obstetrician who dealt with difficult pregnancies even though the only difficulty with mine was that I was HIV-positive. I was really upset by the way I was treated. I think he had decided because I was positive that I must be a junkie mother. I felt that the whole time I saw him during that pregnancy he was judging me and not listening to things I wanted because he knew better than me, which frustrated me, because I'd put a lot of time and thought into the pregnancy. It was extremely important to me and I wanted to do everything I could to make it the best it possibly could be.

Even with the advancements in treatments, not all women find their doctors supportive of their desires to become mothers. Janice, 26, and diagnosed 10 years before the interview, had to seek the opinion of several doctors before she found support for her desire to become a mother.

I've always thought that I'd never, ever have a kid, and different doctors always said, 'No, don't.' Then I moved and I was seeing another doctor there and I asked him about it, because I got with Phillip and he said, 'No, you shouldn't really risk it.' But I just think men don't understand what it's like to have a baby. Like, when you were a kid and how you always thought you will have a baby, and they will be just like you and all that kind of stuff. Then when I moved again I was talking to my [new] doctor about it and he said, 'Yeah, well, there's no reason why not, as long as you look after yourself.' I had to start treatment [to reduce the risk of HIV transmission from mother to baby] when I was twenty weeks and I had to have a caesarean and I couldn't breastfeed, the baby had to have formula, all that type of stuff. So me and Phillip just decided to try and have a baby, and we did!

The [other] doctors were saying, 'Oh, maybe you should just wait a few more years, because treatments will be better then and your viral load is a little bit high, so maybe you shouldn't because that's more risk for the baby.' They made me feel that if I did do it, it was my fault if I put the baby at risk. But my current doctor said that the risk is around 2 percent chance if you do everything they say. Then my viral load went down to undetectable so that was less than a 2 percent chance of the baby having it.

Over the last ten years the advancements in both medicine and knowledge have led to considerable improvements in the experiences of pregnancy and birth for many HIV-positive women. This is particularly evident in the stories told by women who have had more than one child since they were diagnosed.

Layla's first baby was born in 1994:

I had a very long and difficult labour. In the labour ward everything seemed to be fine and not unusual at all – not that I knew, as a first pregnancy – what it should be like. But after I delivered her she was taken away to the nursery and I assumed that was because of the AZT and that they wanted to monitor her while they were giving her the AZT, but I felt like I had no control over that at all, and that I couldn't say, 'Is that what should happen? Is that what usually happens?' I was put back in a room with three other women who had their babies with them, which was very difficult, and there were only curtains between the women. There was a communal waste bag for sheets and towels, but I was told that I couldn't use it. I had a special one next to my bed with this yellow 'Contaminated Waste' bag in it. All over my folder there were yellow stickers and when I went to the nursery I noticed they were putting gloves on to change my baby's nappy, which they were not doing for other babies. I think I was just so overwhelmed by having a baby in that whole situation that I couldn't challenge anything then. I noticed every time I went to the nursery to feed the baby I felt like I was having to educate the nurses so that I was being treated like a human being, otherwise they were making assumptions about who I was and what my life was like.

Layla had her second child in 2001:

I had [my second baby] at the [same hospital] again and they were wonderful. I felt like my status wasn't an issue at all. This time when I was offered my own room I said, 'Yes, thank you, for as long as possible!' They just were wonderful and they went out of their way to be helpful. I noticed when I went to the first appointment at the hospital they brought out my old file and it still had yellow stickers on it, but nothing like that happened during this pregnancy at all. They went as far as not keeping the charts at the end of the bed so they were not there for everyone to see. So they were really quite conscious of my privacy and confidentiality and I think it really helped having the paediatric HIV service so close to the hospital. So they were liaising more closely and regularly, I suppose. This time the baby was with me the whole time, which makes sense if I am going to be administering AZT when I go home. You would think they would want you to do it while you're there to get used to it. But I just think that with my first baby, people were really judgemental about someone's status, and if you are positive it's because you're a specific type of person.

Despite the initial opposition, the stigma and the worry, the women in this study who pursued motherhood described it as an incredible and amazing experience. Their feelings are captured in the words of Stephanie, who was 33 and diagnosed three years at the time of interview, and told by her first doctor that she should focus on her health rather than becoming a mother:

For me it has been a really wonderful experience that I thought I would have to forgo. It's all beautiful; the best experience of my life has been to have my baby.

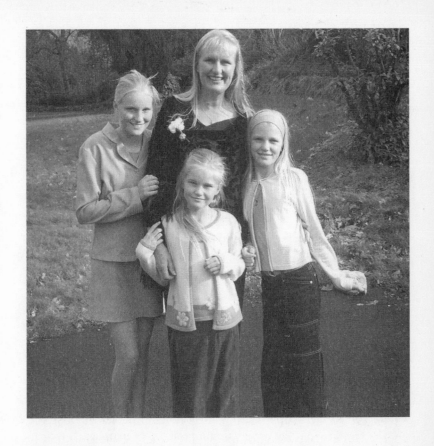

Johanne Greally

Johanne Greally lives in Wellington, New Zealand. Formerly a research technician studying reproductive physiology, she is now an Honours Law student intending to specialise in the fields of medicine, human rights and disability rights. When not studying, lobbying, renovating, or doing 'girl things' with her daughters, her uncanny knack for being 'on the spot' by chance adds to her collection of Police Commendations.

Johanne Greally

MY CHILDREN HAVE
COMPENSATED ME TENFOLD

I have had what I consider to be five miracle babies, born through significant adversity and suffering: John, who I was told would put me in a wheelchair; Catherine, conceived after years of infertility; Petra, who was seven months in utero when a quirky accident left me with a broken pelvis; Elizabeth, conceived after the miscarriage of her brother Michael and whose father walked out when I was three months pregnant with her; and finally, Luke, whose twin Grace did not make it, but who was born after seven months of indescribable agony so great I couldn't walk for most of the pregnancy.

All of them have been worth the pain. Pain is finite. It pauses when you sleep; stops when you recover. But set against the cherished beauty of each of my babies – each of them so totally different but so infinitely loveable – the pain is forgotten. Each child has compensated me tenfold for all I've been through.

My story begins when I was twelve and a student at a small school in the Kaimai Ranges of New Zealand. In our physical education class one day we were playing netball. I was goalshooter, where my height would aid me but where I wouldn't get in the way of the better players. Surprisingly, I shot a goal just as the full-time whistle went and everyone started moving back to the classroom. I stood stock still in the position I had landed in after shooting the goal, terrified of moving or even calling out. The bolt of pain I felt on landing was incomprehensible. The teacher and children had disappeared inside when, thankfully, one child came back because she had forgotten her sandals. 'What are you doing still here?' she asked. 'I can't move,' I whispered, fearing if I talked more loudly I would receive another searing dose of pain.

The teacher and the class returned and stood around looking at me standing like a statue frozen in the middle of a turn. I couldn't understand why the teacher had not called an ambulance, because it was obvious to me that I had broken my back. 'Move your arms down,' he said, and to my surprise I found I could move my arms down. 'Now move your leg forward.' Why would he tell me to do that, and where was the stretcher, and didn't he know that paralysed people shouldn't move? I said nothing and gritted my teeth and moved my leg one step forward. He then told me to move the next leg, and guided me like a remote control robot into school where I waited for my mother to come. I felt really stupid. Here I was saying that I couldn't move and then being able to step all the way to the classroom. Maybe the other kids thought I was being melodramatic and exaggerating, which was certainly not something approved of in this country school where pain, endurance and toughness were much-admired traits.

Scheurmann's disease affects the growth of the endplates of the vertebrae, causing them to become softer and misshapen. As a result, the bones in the spine become wedge-shaped. And that's what I was told I had.

I hated pain, as I suppose most people do. But even more I hated my incapacity. I always felt a rush to get things done, because the next day my back could go, and I would be unable to do the simplest things. Still, at seventeen I somehow managed to leave home and moved from Kaimai, 500 km down to Wallaceville on the outskirts of Wellington, where I joined the reproductive physiology team at Wallaceville Research Centre as a trainee technician. But without the immediate support of my family I found life very difficult. When my back went out and I was unable to move, I had no one to rely on. I even had to ask one of my male flatmates to buy me some tampons one day because I couldn't get out of bed.

I tried all sorts of cures and methods to relieve the pain and reduce my incapacity. Sometimes I could do almost anything, including partying and dancing all night; other times I spent weeks on end going to hospital every morning before work and spending an hour in traction to try to get some relief. I tried different herbal remedies, drugs and painkillers; my use of the latter skyrocketed. I went to a chiropractor. The other patients sat around the outside of the waiting room as I hung from the door frame unable to sit down, and unable to stop the tears falling from my eyes. When the next patient's name was called, those waiting decided – unanimously – that I should be the one to go next. The chiropractor twisted and cracked my neck, which seemed strange, when the pain was in my back. About a week later I was pruning a tree when my neck cracked by itself. What had really cracked was one of the discs, and I ended up in a neck brace for eight weeks. I did not know whether it was the chiropractor who had caused this new problem, whether it was a natural progression or whether I was just susceptible to neck injury due to my misshapen spine. From then on I regularly had cracked discs (sometimes called slipped discs or bulging discs) in my neck as well as in my back.

At work I fought to be able to rent one of the single men's huts which were cheap accommodation for male employees only. In 1979 women government employees were not allowed the same privileges as men – until someone stood up and changed things and I eventually moved in.

Along with struggling to get through each day with the constant fear of further deterioration, I worried about getting a house, having a family and securing my future – afraid of one day being alone and incapacitated. On the day I started work I took out a home ownership account and began saving towards my first house. At the age of 20, and with help from my parents, I became the owner of a small home in the centre of town about ten minutes from work.

Not long after, I met Peter. He worked at the local bottle store and was full of a lot of talk but sadly, very little action. His family were locals and he had nine sisters. The best thing about him was his family, who were so welcoming and caring. When he asked me to marry him I said yes without a lot of thought. I was extremely optimistic that with the good financial foundation I had provided and the values he must have assimilated from his family, that even if I did end up in a wheelchair eventually, we would never be starving or out on the street. I was really young and, in my naïveté, believed that someone from such a stable upbringing would settle down.

Unfortunately, to Peter, money was like water. Being in debt was never a problem because there was always another day to pay it off. Because of my disease he assumed that we would not have children or maybe just one. He did not reckon with my deep determination to overcome all obstacles to have children. Peter didn't tell me he didn't really want children at all, having had enough of his younger sisters and being loath to have a baby in his room ever again. On top of that, he did not like working and was unable to hold down a job for any length of time. He would say it was his parents' fault for not letting him leave school to take up a trade, or his employers' fault for not recognising his talents. Later it became my fault for not selling my house to provide him with capital for his own business. Later still, it was the fault of his children for existing and thereby reducing our earnings as I cared for them.

But my skeletal frailty caused me to want to hurry and have children, to achieve what I could as soon as possible. I was wanting to try for children before my frame could not bear the possibility of a child.

I found out I was pregnant while on holiday, when I was 22. I had suspected I might be before we left even though the home pregnancy kit had given the thumbs down. As we were going to a three-day rock concert at Sweetwaters, I had another test, which to my joy was positive. I rushed down to my grandmother's house to tell her. Peter and I continued on to the concert. I was ill with morning sickness and Peter was drunk and violent. At one stage he lent on the middle pole of my brother's tent which collapsed as I cringed in the corner trying to hide. Later he came back to try and find me, but I kept very quiet as he cursed and swore. At the time I never put the two facts together: that Peter was now a father and that he was behaving atrociously. What I did know, though, was that I was no longer the happy party girl.

On returning home I went to see my doctor. I was totally unprepared for his reaction. 'There will be no problem getting you an abortion,' he said. 'You meet all the requirements on both physical and mental grounds.' 'But,' I stammered, 'I don't want an abortion. I want a baby.' I felt shocked, belittled and disempowered by him.

'Your back is unable to support just you, let alone a baby. You will never be able to carry a baby. You will be in a wheelchair by the time you are seven months.' It was true that my back couldn't support me at that time, and I had been trussed up in a corset-type back-brace off and on for over a year, so that I could not move around freely even without a baby. What would happen when I couldn't rely on my stomach muscles to take some weight?

But the word 'abortion' had brought forth an instinctual protective response from deep within, a response from a mother who had accepted there was already a baby growing inside and who needed her. My baby was a present fact, not a promise or a threat. The doctor didn't know me. He didn't even ask me what I wanted. Despite my determination to overcome my physical disability, the doctor left me feeling less capable and fearful – fearful for my baby and my future.

My courage could have engendered a certain respect and support from my workmates, but the all-day morning sickness and tiredness I was suffering led me to be seen as the worker who had rapidly exhausted her sick leave, was barely 'present' when at work anyway, and had let the team down. I was so worried about how I would keep things together.

I was about three months pregnant when I started noticing that I could move more easily. I ditched the back-brace as my tummy grew, and I found that I could now bend forward a little. I became less cautious about my movements, not experiencing the usual jolt of pain whenever I twisted suddenly.

Meanwhile, Peter had decided he wanted to be self-employed. I suggested buying a burger bar and working it up into a restaurant when we had some money saved. 'There is no way you will ever, ever, see me stoop as low as to work in a burger bar,' Peter replied. He was adamant: 'It's a restaurant or nothing.' A small restaurant came up for sale in Featherston. I borrowed money and we bought it.

All through the pregnancy my back continued to improve. I was now able to lift and bend, even chop wood by the time I was at the seven-month mark. In addition to my full-time employment at the research station and the restaurant in the evenings, I was also organising a catering service most weekends.

Years later, my curiosity about how my pregnancy could have relieved so many of the symptoms I was experiencing was satisfied at a group physiotherapy session. A woman with the same problem told me she had seen a top specialist in England who had recommended she become pregnant. The specialist had found many of his women patients had improved substantially but did not know whether the change was due to altered posture or was hormonally influenced. I attended the physiotherapy because an X-ray revealed I also had Perthe's disease (similar to Scheurmann's disease, but affecting the hip joint rather than the spine). This extra condition had been masked by the Scheurmann's disease and the hip pain I felt had, until then, been thought to be referred pain from my spine. Although I am now susceptible to having disc problems, have wedge-shaped vertebrae and have bouts of back pain, following John's birth I never again experienced anywhere near the degree of incapacity or pain.

John was born naturally in a small rural hospital. Being his mother was everything I hoped for. I loved everything about him. I loved sitting with my face in his hair just smelling him. I spent hours talking to him. He always appeared to understand me.

Unfortunately we had to close our restaurant and sell it for a loss. This meant I had to return to work when John was only three months old. I missed him badly. No one who had taken maternity leave had returned before, and given the work record of my last few months there, it was understandable that I wasn't welcomed back with open arms. Although I wanted more children, I thought it best that all our debts be cleared first. Foolishly I had an injection of Depo Provera, not realising and not being informed of the side-effects or possible consequences. As a result it was four years before I became pregnant with Catherine.

After another pregnancy with all-day morning sickness, I gave up full-time work and within two years was pregnant with Petra. The doctor knew better than to threaten my babies this time. (When, a couple of years afterwards, I went to see him after learning that my baby had died in utero, I had decided I was going to hit the next medical professional who minimised my loss by calling my dead baby a 'non-viable foetus'.) I was tensed up, just in case he did, when he came and hugged me and told me how very, very sorry he was and then let me cry and cry for my baby.

In July 1990, I was seven months pregnant with Petra, and on a fine winter's day – after days of rain – I decided to take my children and some others after school to feed the ducks. Catherine had just turned two and with us was her adorable 18-month-old friend Amy. The older children headed for the playground as I went with the two little ones towards the lake. Catherine started squealing as a big goose attempted to take the bread from her hand. While I bent over her trying to get her to release the bread, Amy continued toddling towards the lake. Even though absorbed with rescuing Catherine, I did not for one moment take my eye off Amy, and made a mental calculation of how fast she could toddle in her gumboots, and at what point I would have to race to intercept her if she kept heading for the lake. As if in slow motion, she suddenly tripped on a pebble and cartwheeled perfectly a number of times and disappeared off the edge. I bolted to the edge with my heart hammering as I heard the splash, praying desperately that she would be floating. I looked over into a dark green soupy lake with the terrifying realisation that I could see nothing. I felt like crying and vomiting and screaming. I thought I glimpsed, in a split second, Amy's orange and purple pompom hat way under the surface.

I knew I had to jump in. I had no idea how deep it was, I so much hoped it would be shallow enough for me to find her, but deep enough that my unborn baby and I would not be badly injured. I felt a searing bolt of pain as I landed in waist-deep water, reached out and found Amy. She coughed and began breathing almost the instant that I brought her to the surface. I tore her clothes off and shoved her down the front of my top to warm her.

The bottom of the lake was formed with large rocks, not the sand or mud I had half expected, so my feet had landed at funny angles. I attempted to move one of my legs and screamed in pain. I had no idea what my injury was but knew that I was trapped standing in the lake. My boots were full of water and lifting my feet out of them was impossible. The joint holding my pelvis together (symphisis pubis) had broken and every time I attempted to lift a leg the ends of the bones ground against each other. (Later, an X-ray would show the end of the pubic ramsis had also fractured.) I took a deep breath and pulled my leg forward. I screamed again. If it had not been for the necessity to keep Amy warm and dry, I would have lain down in the water and used my arms to pull me out.

It was only a matter of weeks till Petra was due. Fearful that any major medical or surgical interventions could harm her, I instead decided to use a special belt to hold the bones together while putting Catherine in care until Petra was born. Peter had been unemployed again for a year but was not prepared to assist in any significant way. The six weeks till her birth were a painful blur, but thankfully my pelvic bones began knitting back together not long after she was born. Petra had suffered no harm in the accident and was the sweetest little baby. She and I are extremely close; even now, fourteen years later, she admits that she tells me everything. I have always been able to tell, even from a distance, if she is in some sort of trouble.

When I had recovered I began to have more involvement in the community. I joined a human rights organisation and a group to help women who had problems during pregnancy, which I found to be really rewarding. I felt I was contributing to society. I stopped relying on Peter for anything. I expected nothing in the way of physical or financial support.

I was delighted when I found out that I was pregnant with Elizabeth, which came within a month of my previous baby's miscarrying and of me developing pelvic inflammatory disease (PID). I had been told at the hospital that it would be unlikely I would have another baby at all given the extent of the PID. They also told me I shouldn't have any more, regardless.

Peter left when I was about three months pregnant. He made it clear that he had never wanted children, he had wanted a working wife and a house in Karori where the rich people live. A month later he left for Greece with his girlfriend.

I kept away from anyone I thought would be negative about the baby. This did not stop the neighbour who had comforted me when I miscarried with, 'It's just as well, as you would never have coped with four children,' from this time offering the advice: 'You will have to do something about that as soon as possible because you wouldn't cope with having another baby by yourself.'

In contrast, I had friends who rallied around and really helped and did not see my decision to continue my pregnancy as stupid and selfish. A fellow pregnancy counsellor even took the children for a weekend every fortnight. As my weakened pelvic joint started pulling apart later in pregnancy, friends came to help with the housework. A friend, John, from Wellington, came out every fortnight to mow my lawn and took young John under his wing.

Later in the pregnancy a woman called Mary, who I had met once in Wellington, took leave from her job in Dunedin and moved in with us. She took charge of the meals, children and the whole household and stayed until Elizabeth was a month old. I will never forget her kindness. Elizabeth's birth was like a party, with eleven of us present for the occasion.

Elizabeth was my biggest baby. She was chubby and round and never stopped smiling. Now at 11 she is so even-tempered and responsible. She is not fazed by anything.

John (my lawn mower friend) asked me to marry him when Elizabeth was 4, two years after Peter divorced me. The sorting of the previous matrimonial property was still not finished. Under New Zealand law each party gets half the house no matter who bought it, and each party is responsible for half the debt no matter who acquired it.

John obtained a new job so that he could support his new large family; previously he had been working mostly unpaid for a charitable organisation.

We looked forward to having children and hoped that if I had any more problems, with John's presence and salary we would be able to afford someone to help me. Only a month after we were married we were delighted to discover I was pregnant again. My pregnancy started pretty much as normal. My delight quickly turned to 'Oh no, here we go again!' as the first of many waves of nausea struck.

I was 10 weeks pregnant when my waters broke. I knew from the volume of fluid that the baby didn't stand a chance. The next day I went for a scan and we couldn't believe our eyes when we saw that I had been having twins and one was still moving and swimming about. The second sac had ruptured. Luke's placenta was torn, with blood still leaking out of it, but he was holding on and his little arms and legs were waving away.

About two weeks after this I noticed something was wrong with my pelvis. Little twinges when I put weight on each leg when walking soon became bigger twinges, and a week later it was not only walking that was painful, but sitting and standing as well. The doctor referred me to a physiotherapist and applied to the Accident Compensation Corporation (ACC) for some home-help. My central pelvic joint had broken again; it had never healed properly after my accident at the lake. This meant that if I was upright (even sitting slightly upright) my weight combined with the weight of the baby would force the bones apart. If I moved in any other way then nerves would be trapped between the bones as the ends of the bones ground past each other. What followed was, without doubt, the worst six months of my life. Every day was a day of pain. Even rolling from one side of the bed to the other was a nightmare. Most of my day was spent lying in bed. The more upright I was, the greater the pain in my pelvis, but the flatter I lay, the worse the nausea and the heartburn became. Whether or not to slide up or down the bed a few inches when the pain at one end became too intense, formed a continuous calculation that occupied my day.

No amount of belts and bindings would stabilise my pelvis. Crutches had helped me walk to some extent initially, but after a while trying to balance solely on one crutch and then the other caused strains in my shoulder muscles, and they would spasm. To get to physiotherapy to treat my shoulders involved getting to the car, getting into the car and putting a strap around my leg so that I could lift my leg from the accelerator and move it to the brake if I needed to slow down. The seat had to be as flat as possible but still allow me to see over the dashboard. After a while I ceased going to the physiotherapist or doctor and only went out when there was an emergency with one of the children or when the ACC unhelpfully demanded I did.

I couldn't use a wheelchair for two reasons. If I sat upright, gravity and the baby would push the bones apart which would also cause movement in the sacroiliac joints where the pelvic bones attach to the spine. It took a bone graft and a later fusion to stop the continuous background ache from the sacroiliac joints. Even if I had been able to sit, I would not have been able to move the wheel with my arms. A kindly occupational therapist brought me a small trolley – against hospital regulations – on which I could put my chest and arms and then propel myself forward by squiggling my toes. This was a huge improvement on the crutches, and caused far less damage to my shoulders.

As time progressed, John became more reluctant to return home each night at a reasonable time. He did not like strangers present in the house, and with me so often absent in the bedroom was not always sure how to cope with the older children. We did not know then that John had Asperger's Syndrome – an inherited genetic disability which, among other more significant charac-teristics, unhelpfully led him to prefer to avoid difficult social or pressured situations at all costs. He felt his home 'invaded' by helpers and just wanted to be hidden away from it all. He was also working longer hours, not only to make up for the slowness that comes with his disability at times, but also to try to help us get ahead financially by exceeding sales targets. He would come home quite exhausted.

The most help I received came from a mentally ill couple from down the road whose own children had been removed by the authorities.

The physical pain was only part of the problem. The emotional angst of what was happening to my family and my home was extreme. I, the mother and wife, was unable to care for my family. My children could attend none of their regular activities, and the girls were infested with head lice. I was extremely worried that their father would find out how bad things were and try to seek permanent custody, an option that I saw as being extremely detrimental to them all. Elizabeth, especially, did not know her father and had had nothing to do with him. She would suffer home sickness if we were apart more than a couple of days.

We were entitled to no help from the state as my incapacity was from an injury and when that is the case the ACC is legally obliged to provide all support needed. This is why the hospital could not help in providing equipment. Unfortunately, their position became very clear from the first visit by their so-called independent professional assessors – who included, I'm sorry to say, women. 'How do we know that this is really from an injury?' they asked. 'What proof have you got that this is not just a pregnancy-related condition?' I refused to have X-rays or allow any diagnostic technique or treatment that would harm my baby, and I felt this was being used against me. 'It is *your* choice to continue with this pregnancy – Why should ACC pay for your choices?' Next they questioned the extent of my disability: 'If you really are as sick as you say you are, then you should be in hospital.' They actually laughed when I described my transport difficulties: 'Let us know when you go out so we won't be on the road.'

They also required me to go to Wellington to see a specialist from Australia, knowing full well that I had no way to get to Wellington, and the enormous amount of pain I would be in just getting out to a taxi. Finally they made the completely insane determination that an at-home mother of four does five hours of work a week. They were so condescending, calling me 'Dear', and making it clear they thought I was stupid for continuing my pregnancy, stupid for not using sufficient quantities of pain-killers, and exaggerating the amount of pain and disability suffered. To them I was no more than an unpaid incompetent mother.

One of the reasons I was so stunned, I suppose, was that almost all the women I had known and associated with were empathetic and supportive of other women. This was especially so when I lived in a small rural town where there was much poverty and violence. The women there relied heavily on solidarity, the friendly support and comfort of each other. This was the first time I had seen women in a position of power (for in the end they determined to a large extent the amount of extra suffering I had to endure) use their position to unfairly abuse and cause harm to another woman. If there ever had been pressure to abort it was from these women.

Crying was no good; if it involved sobbing, it only created more pain. I learnt to cry with just my eyes and my mind. I talked to my baby and told him how much I loved him and that I would never let anyone hurt him. I was so conscious of him and because I was so still, felt his every movement. Sometimes it seemed that it was just me and him against the world, that we were both on the same team, fighting for the same thing and together we would win – the successful prize being his safe delivery.

I used to talk to him about all sorts of things. With the baby that I had miscarried, I remember talking to him and telling him out loud how much I loved him. I was so grateful that I had done that before finding out his heartbeat had stopped. Afterward it became important to me that he had known that he was loved before he died. I hadn't talked to the other babies like that. When I was pregnant with Elizabeth I had been so busy and so distressed that I hadn't had as much time to communicate with her, but with Luke I had every hour of every day.

Often when John came home from work at night he would lift me into our swimming pool so I could have a relatively pain-free break. I would lock my knees together and kick with my feet. This would relieve some of the terrible cramping in my legs. The horrible thing was when the swim came to an end and I had to face the full effects of gravity again. I can understand how astronauts returning to earth must feel.

Because I had spent my whole pregnancy on my side, the baby was lying transverse or breach. It was looking more likely that I would have a caesarean. I had taken part in a large and heated public debate with the only obstetrician in the region who would turn a baby, and if I had a caesarean then he would be the one to do it; I just did not want to be in the same room as him, let alone have my baby's life in his hands. We looked up on the internet to discover methods of turning babies, and my midwife found some very improbable exercises to do. We tried doing some strange things in the pool to get the baby to turn and were getting more desperate as his due date passed. In the end, I applied an icepack just below my ribs and ate a heap of ice. Boy, did he move! Boy, did it hurt! He seemed to stretch sideways. (I have since found out this can be dangerous as a baby can end up wrapping the cord around his or her neck.) I had a scan the next day and when he was found to be in the normal position they induced me straight away in case he should turn again.

I spent my labour in a large bath and Luke was born naturally. I had worried about how the amounts of pain I had been in would affect his endocrine system, but he seemed fine after getting off to a very slow start.

Luke has since been diagnosed with high functioning autism, which I think is probably a matter of genetics rather than the effects of the pregnancy. He has incredible potential and is always surprising us with some new knowledge he has gained. He loves the program *Decisive Battles* on the History Channel and for his sixth birthday recently asked for a book on Egyptian mythology. I can never remember him being disobedient (even as a 2-year-old), and he just loves doing things to please his parents and teachers.

After I had recovered sufficiently, I filed a court action against the way the ACC had treated me and while I won on two of the grounds, I lost on the two grounds that were most important: how much work a woman at home does, and what it is worth. This was a test case. At issue was the question of the minimum amount of input required to adequately provide physically for a family of six. I took the case to appeal, not for me personally but because the state should not be able to say that any mother at home only does between $5^{1}/_{4}$ and $5^{1}/_{2}$ hours work per week.

After winning the appeal I started studying for a law degree. I am now at Victoria University studying towards my LLB

Honours. In November 2004 I had another operation which has enabled me to walk – and sometimes run – on my own.

For many pregnant women, life is made harder by the view that pregnancy is the equivalent of a self-inflicted injury and the recipient got what they deserved for the choices they made.

What pregnant women need to hear is that they are living out the most marvellous and creative power for good. I look at my beautiful daughters and hope they enjoy motherhood as much as I do and that their circumstances and health enable them to be supported through pregnancy and enjoy their families.

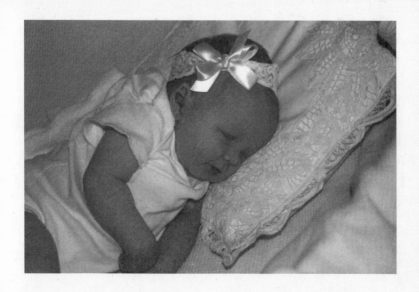

Heather Arnold

Heather Arnold lives in St. Louis, Missouri, USA. She enjoys scrapbooking and talking long-distance to her best friend, Tanya. She takes pride in being the wife of a US Army Combat Medic. She loves to travel and recently visited Morocco. The only thing she likes more than being a mom, is being a mom of three.

Heather Arnold

THE 'STANDARD OF CARE' WOULD BE
TO ABORT MY UNBORN CHILD

'This is nothing short of a miracle.' Those were the words of my perinatologist, months after she advised me to terminate my pregnancy.

At the age of 18, I was diagnosed with Mixed Connective Tissue Disease (MCTD), an auto-immune disorder that is similar to rheumatoid arthritis and lupus. This disease left me struggling to do simple everyday things like pouring a glass of milk or brushing my hair. My rheumatologist began a series of medications that helped me cope with the pain and stiffness that accompanies MCTD. Gradually I was able to regain control of my life and look forward. When I was 20, I married my high school sweetheart – the man who had been by my side from the signs of the first symptom through the diagnosis and to the adjustment of a life-changing illness. We were anxious to start a family, fearing the unknown factors of this changing disease and not wanting to miss our window of opportunity to have a child. In October 1999 I became pregnant.

I will never forget how excited I was to call my rheumatologist and tell her the good news of our expected arrival. Nor will I ever forget the paralysing fear and pain that came with her response. She explained that she had just received the results of my recent pulmonary functions test, a test that I have routinely for MCTD, and the results showed that I had pulmonary hypertension. I was stunned at this news. I didn't feel sick. I wasn't having a hard time breathing. I didn't understand what this meant. Then she informed me that being pregnant would only worsen my condition and that the 'standard of care' would be to abort my unborn child. She recommended that I go to a perinatologist instead of a basic obstetrician/gynaecologist, and that I should seek treatment immediately.

I was sent to a perinatologist with a wonderful reputation. She was very cut-and-dried and did not sugar-coat my situation at all. She simply pulled out her medical books and showed me case studies of women with pulmonary hypertension who were pregnant. We read over them together, case by case. The best prognosis she could give me was a 50 percent chance of surviving the pregnancy. She could not begin to speculate on any prognosis for my child. She explained that I would be hospitalised through-out most of the pregnancy and on a ventilator. Pulmonary hypertension occurs when the blood pressure in the pulmonary artery rises significantly, causing shortness of breath, fainting, dizziness, and other symptoms. The added pressure of a baby pressing on my lungs would cause more problems. This doctor also reinforced that the 'standard of care' in my condition would be to abort the baby. I told her immediately that abortion was not an option and that I would be carrying this baby as long as I possibly could. She encouraged me to go home and talk with my husband before making the decision, although my mind was already made up.

My husband was completely supportive of my decision, also agreeing that abortion was not the right answer. My family stood by my side and supported my decision to carry this baby. The only opposition came from my father-in-law. While he understood my desire to have a baby, he was more concerned about his son facing the possibility of becoming a widower and possibly a single father at the age of 21. He wanted to protect my husband from the pain that my death would bring, and I understood that. I was also concerned about how my husband would cope if tragedy did strike. If our child survived and I did not, what would he tell the baby? How could he explain the love I had for this child? So, I began keeping a journal, a love letter, of sorts, to our baby. And our friends, family and many others started praying.

Ten weeks after I found out I was pregnant I was sent to take another series of pulmonary tests so my doctors could track the progression of the hypertension. They were baffled by the results – the pulmonary hypertension no longer existed. They couldn't explain it. There is no known cure for this condition and it can't go away on its own. 'This is nothing short of a miracle,' was the only response any of my doctors could offer.

During an ultrasound a few weeks later, choroid plexus cysts were found on my baby's brain. I was not given much information about them. I was only told that they could either go away or they could be signs of developmental anomalies, in which case, again, the 'standard of care' would be to abort. Six weeks later, at the next ultrasound, the cysts were gone.

On 25 June 2000, I gave birth to a beautiful, red-headed baby girl, who is perfect in every way. We named her Miracle. Five years later, Miracle now has two little brothers.

Our oldest son, Riley, was also found to have choroid plexus cysts and we were again reminded of the 'standard of care'. Today, he is a curious 4-year-old. Before our youngest son Joey was born, I was diagnosed with lupus. He was born three weeks early via emergency c-section due to a 60 percent placental abruption – a common effect of lupus. Thanks to the quick thinking of my doctor, both he and I survived without complications.

With all three pregnancies I chose to stop taking my medication because it can cause cleft lip in unborn children. I was blessed with fewer pains and less stiffness during my pregnancies and did not notice the lack of medication. I am so glad that I didn't go along with what everyone told me was the 'standard of care' for my babies.

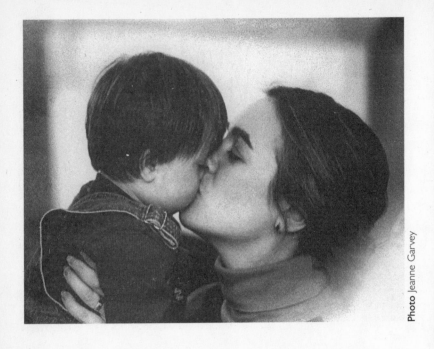

Elizabeth R. Schiltz

Elizabeth Schiltz is an Associate Professor of Law at the University of St. Thomas School of Law in Minneapolis, Minnesota, USA. She teaches Contracts, Banking Law, Sales and Credit and Payment Devices. She is married to another law professor, Patrick Schiltz, and is the proud mother of Anna, Joseph, Peter, and Katherine.

Elizabeth R. Schiltz

LIVING IN THE SHADOW OF MÖNCHBERG

I was born and raised in Germany. My father was drafted into the US Army during World War II, sent over to England with the US Field Artillery, fought his way through the D-Day invasion and the Ardennes, and was finally mustered out in Paris when the war ended. He stayed in Europe as a civilian working for the US Army. Family legend has it that he used the free call given to all US soldiers at the end of the war to call my mom in Pittsburgh, and ask her to marry him and join him in Germany. That is where they lived until my father retired and they moved back to Pittsburgh.

To get the German economy back on its feet after the war, the Army subsidized the hiring of Germans to help the Americans as handymen, maids or nannies. One of the people that my parents hired to help with our rapidly growing family was a woman named Theresa Böhm. She was initially hired as a maid, then became more of a nanny, and eventually became a cherished unofficial member of our family. I knew her only as Oma – grandma. She was our substitute German grandma, filling in for the ones living an ocean away from us. She was the one whose musty little home we visited on holidays and in whose huge feather bed we snuggled in long visits during summer vacations.

Oma was born in a little village near the town of Hadamar. Hadamar sits in the shadow of a tall hill called Mönchberg – Monk's Mountain. On top of that hill stands an old Franciscan monastery, which was converted into a state hospital and nursing home in 1803. In 1940, however, that hospital was turned into one of the infamous Nazi 'killing centers'.[1] These were the six institutions spread all over Germany where first children, and later also adults, with disabilities such as (in the language of those times) 'idiocy and mongolism (especially when associated with blindness and deafness), microcephaly, hydrocephaly, malformations of all kinds, especially of limbs, head, and spinal column, and paralysis, including spastic conditions'[2] were taken, systematically starved to death or gassed, and cremated.[3]

Oma rarely spoke to us about her experiences during the war. But we know that she was affected by the experience of living in the shadow of Mönchberg. All the accounts one reads about the Hadamar Institute emphasize the heavy smoke from the crematorium chimneys, visible to the local inhabitants, and horrid in smell.[4] One contemporary account of the effect of living with that smoke is found in a letter written in August 1941 by the Bishop of Limburg:

> The effect of the principles at work here is that children call each other names and say, 'You're crazy; you'll be sent to the baking oven in Hadamar.' . . . You hear old folks say, 'Don't send me to a State hospital! When the feeble-minded have been finished off, the next useless eaters whose turn will come are the old people.'[5]

Oma was always terrified of hospitals. As she grew older, she had increasingly emphatic conversations with my mother about not letting anyone take her to a hospital if she got sick.

I was the fifth of sixth children. Oma loved us all very dearly, but she had a favorite, and she never made even the feeblest attempt to hide it. The other five of us were all her *Silberfische* – silverfishes. My older brother, Jim, was her *Goldfisch* – her goldfish.

Jim was born mentally retarded. When he was born back in 1952, the medical professionals counselled my parents to send him to live in an institution. My parents refused, and with much work and love, they taught Jim to do all those things that the medical professionals told my parents he would never do, like talk and walk. Jim graduated from high school. He is bilingual – fluent in German as well as English. He reads the newspaper every day. Jim has held the same full-time position in the kitchen of a country club for twenty years now, and does not receive any sort of public assistance. Jim is known around our family as 'the human juke-box', for his uncanny ability to remember the lyrics to any song, from any era, by any artist.

Oma doted on Jim. When he was a baby, she spent endless hours massaging his legs and encouraging him to walk – indeed, she was the first person in our family to see him actually walk on his own. Once Jim got to be 6 or 7 years old, he would spend a couple of weeks every summer with Oma. One of the things she spent a lot of time doing was teaching him fine table manners. If he did something that did not pass her strict standards of etiquette, she would admonish him: *'Wir sind hier bei vornehme Leute!'* – 'We are in the company of distinguished people!' Oma was emphatic that Jim should take his place in society with 'distinguished people', that nothing about his condition justified any sort of exclusion.

In some sense, although we did not live in the town of Hadamar, I think that all the kids in my family grew up in the shadow of Mönchberg as well. I cannot remember a time when I did not know that the first targets of the Nazi's gas chambers were people with disabilities. I cannot remember a time when I did not know that my brother Jim would probably not have been allowed to live if he had been born just ten years earlier, in the same hospital in Frankfurt, Germany, where I was later born – a former German military hospital in which my mother noticed, the first time she was there, swastikas carved in the borders along the top of the walls. I grew up with a visceral awareness of the potential within humanity to decide that it is legitimate to kill certain categories of people because of the costs that their life imposes on society. I grew up loving a brother who I knew was in one of the categories of humans that the Nazis had determined possessed a *lebens-unwertes Leben* – a 'life unworthy of life' – a life whose cost to society exceeded its worth.[6]

But that was years ago and far away, right? I grew up, moved back to the United States for college, went to law school, then plunged into my life as an all-American working mom, practicing law and raising kids in the modern, progressive metropolis of Minneapolis, Minnesota. And then something happened to me, and my life changed, and in so many ways now, on so many days, I feel as though I am still living in the shadow of Mönchberg.

What happened was this. When I was about five months pregnant with my third child, Peter, I got a copy of this:

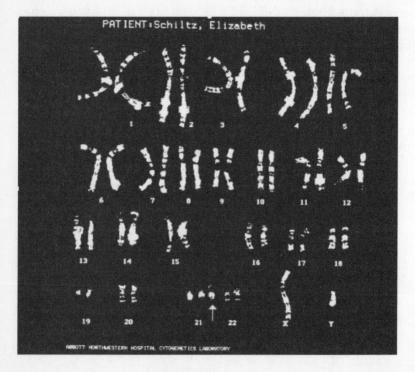

This is the karyotype of one of Petey's cells that was floating in amniotic fluid extracted from my womb by a big needle during an amniocentesis. The arrow in the karyotype points out that Petey's cells have three, rather than the usual two, copies of chromosome number 21. This indicates that he has an incurable chromosomal condition called trisomy 21, or Down syndrome, or, in the old-fashioned language of the Nazi regime, 'mongolism'.

The amniocentesis that my husband and I chose to undergo was the fourth in a series of prenatal tests we had performed during that pregnancy. The first was a blood test to assess the amount of alpha-fetoprotein (AFP) in my blood. That AFP test is routinely offered to pregnant women early in pregnancy, along with a slew of other tests. Every time you go to your doctor when you are pregnant, a nurse seems to take vials of blood to test for things like anemia, Rh factors, HIV – all conditions affecting the mother's health directly, and the baby's health indirectly. With Petey, my AFP test showed a lower-than-normal amount of the alpha-fetoprotein, thus indicating a higher-than-normal statistical probability that the baby I was carrying had Down syndrome. The statistical probability that my baby had Down syndrome, based on my age alone at the time, was 1:378. My AFP test results raised the odds to 1:170.

When my obstetrician shared these results with me, I chose to have another, more detailed, blood test, hoping that I would be reassured that nothing was wrong with the baby. In fact, this second test gave me odds of 1:38. Faced with that information, my husband and I decided to have a level 2 ultrasound, a very detailed ultrasound that might detect some of the heart or stomach abnormalities often associated with Down syndrome. Despite the fact that the analysis of that ultrasound showed no signs of Down syndrome, we chose to proceed with the amniocentesis that resulted in that karyotype.

The medical professionals I was dealing with through all those tests were not trying to find information to help me protect the health of my baby. Unlike the tests for anemia or HIV, there is little that can be done about the conditions that these tests were attempting to identify. These tests were offered for the purpose of bestowing upon me a special societal privilege to choose to abort my baby. That karyotype could have been my ticket to a guilt-free, utterly justified, absolutely legal abortion – even that late in my pregnancy. If the technology had existed in the 1940s, that karyotype would almost certainly have been a ticket to Hadamar.

As someone who has always been pro-life, I did not accept these tests for the purpose of obtaining that 'privilege'. I just wanted to *know*, partly in the vain hope that I could be reassured nothing was wrong, but also so that if I could not be reassured, I could at least be prepared. I am a nerd; if I was going to have a baby with Down syndrome, I wanted to read every possible book on the subject before the baby came.

Experiencing this testing sequence first hand, however, gave me some personal insights into the potentially pernicious effects of the prenatal testing process. The tests are all offered in the guise of 'reassurance', along with a battery of other tests.[7] All of these tests carry with them the implication that the responsible mother can and should do something constructive with the results: take extra iron if she is found to be anemic; take AZT if she has HIV; or abort the baby if he or she has Down syndrome. If you lack the financial or other resources to raise a child with a disability, you could easily be swayed by an argument that the knowledge you now possess about the child gives you the responsibility to do something constructive to solve the problem, by aborting the child.

Now, this argument could obviously be a powerful incentive for a person to 'choose' to have an abortion. Going through this process personally made me acutely aware of its potential power.

But this was not the aspect of the experience that really surprised me. What really surprised me was that people did not stop making this argument once I rejected it during the testing phase. When I started telling people that the baby I was expecting would have Down syndrome, I had colleagues ask me incredulously, 'Why are you having this baby?' While there was something rather creepy about being asked that question directly – by someone staring at that big belly of mine, while the baby kicked inside – it was still not too difficult for me to deal with. I was comfortable defending my position that I didn't believe in abortion, that I didn't think I did have any choice in this matter; I was still in familiar, pro-life territory.

But I left that familiar territory the moment that Petey was born, and I found, to my great surprise, that society *still* kept asking that question: Why did you have this baby? I have had people react with marked surprise when they hear that I knew Petey would have Down syndrome before he was born. Though they do not ask aloud, you can see the question in their eyes: 'If you knew, why did you have the baby?' What's buried in that question, what's buried deep in their eyes as they ask it, is the perception of my son as 'a choice' – specifically, my choice – rather than as a unique human being, created in God's image, rather than as a fully-fledged member of the human race.

What I see in their eyes is the lingering shadow of Mönchberg that sometimes keeps me awake at night. I worry that the joint availability of tests and abortion seems to be eroding societal consensus about our collective responsibility for vulnerable people – people with disabilities whose conditions were or could have been diagnosed prenatally, or even people born into difficult family situations or social structures. I am very frightened by the emerging attitude that if a woman exercises her 'choice' to have a child who can be identified in advance as 'vulnerable' for some reason, the woman herself bears the responsibility for dealing with that vulnerability.[8] In other words, if the 'cost' of a certain life is going to be more than its 'worth', someone has to make up the deficit. The assumption seems to be that if you 'choose' to impose that cost on society by having a baby you could so easily have aborted, you should pay the price.

Examples of this attitude abound. Bob Edwards, the scientist who created Great Britain's first in vitro fertilization baby, recently gave a speech at an international fertility conference in France in which he expressed just this attitude. He opined: 'Soon it will be a sin of parents to have a child that carries the heavy burden of genetic disease. We are entering a world where we have to consider the quality of our children.'[9] In other words, if we can identify a genetic condition before a child is born, and the parents choose to have the baby anyway, they are committing a sin. They're making a choice that society is going to have to pay for. It is their choice, their sin – they should be the ones to pay.

Let me give you another example. A couple of years ago a woman's prenatal tests showed her baby would be born with cystic fibrosis. When the baby was born, the HMO [health maintenance organization] initially denied medical coverage, since it was born with a 'pre-existing condition'.[10] Although that decision was overturned, this HMO – at least initially – told the woman in essence: *You knew about this condition before the baby was born. You could have prevented this baby from being born. You chose not to. Since you made that choice, you can find a way to pay for it.*[11]

This same attitude lurks behind the increasing number of wrongful birth and wrongful life suits being brought all over the United States.[12] In these suits, parents of children with disabilities (typically Down syndrome) sue medical professionals for failing to correctly diagnose the condition before birth. The parents argue that they would have aborted the children, and thus 'solved' the problem, if they had known about the condition. Since they were not given that option, they should not bear the costs. Instead, the medical professionals who took their choice away from them should pay. In other words, the 'problem' is the fault of some identifiable person – in this case, a medical professional rather than the mother. That person, rather than society at large, should thus bear the cost.

This attitude is taking hold in other countries as well. In England, for example, a recent investigation found that doctors at one of England's leading heart hospitals – the Royal Brompton Hospital – were discriminating against children with Down syndrome. About half of all children with Down syndrome are born with heart defects that can be fatal if not treated, but typically can be relatively easily fixed with surgery. The inquiry did not find that the Brompton hospital doctors were refusing to provide this life-saving heart surgery to children with Down syndrome, or that they failed to perform such surgery with all due care when they undertook it. However, the report found that 'In some cases there was a failure to provide a balanced view of all the options available to the families' of children with Down syndrome. In consultations, parents of children with Down syndrome would essentially be told that the risks of the surgery were not worthwhile. Doctors 'did not focus sufficiently on what was in the best interests of the child as the patient,' but instead tended to stress the burden that the parents would face in caring for such a child.[13]

One of the most frightening aspects of this report is that it found that the doctors were not intentionally discriminating; they were acting in 'good faith', honestly believing they were doing what was in the best interests of these families. These doctors were acting on their professional belief that the cost of this life-saving heart surgery was less justified for a child with Down syndrome than for a child without it. The cost of saving the disabled child's life is not worth the burden that child would impose on society.

This same attitude also underlies the growing trend of creating 'designer babies', by artificially fertilizing embryos and then conducting pre-implantation genetic screening in order to select only the embryos who lack certain problematic genes, are the desired sex or who have certain features, such as bone marrow tissue suitable for transplant to an ill sibling.[14] Garland E. Allen, a historian of science, recently wrote an article in the magazine *Science*, comparing the social conditions that supported the spread of the eugenics movement in the early part of the last century with today's social conditions. In this article, he expressed his fear that the same conditions exist today, and claimed that, 'As health care costs skyrocket, we are coming to accept a bottom-line, cost-benefit analysis of human life.'[15] We can now create 'perfect' babies. We can also abort less than perfect babies. *It is a matter of choice – your choice, Mom. If you choose to keep that less-than-perfect baby, that is your choice, but it is also your problem. You could have solved it for us. You chose not to. You pay for that choice.*

Those who would adhere to a cost-benefit analysis of the lives of people with disabilities have to admit serious problems in determining how such a morally suspect analysis would ever work in practice. There have been calculations of the cost of allowing a child with Down syndrome to be born.[16] Although I am extremely skeptical of such calculations, I suppose, in theory, I could be convinced that some rough economic analysis might allow some generalizations, at least about the financial costs of raising a hypo-thetical typical child with Down syndrome. But what possible criteria could be rationally imposed to quantify the benefit of such a life? Whose calculation of the benefit could one trust? Should we ask the people who really ought to know – people who live with disabilities? Disability rights activists argue that 'Most people with disabilities rate their quality of life as much higher than other people think. People make the decision [to reject embryos] based on a prejudice that having a disability means having a low quality of life.'[17]

Should we ask parents raising children with disabilities? *The child who never grew*, by Pulitzer and Nobel prize-winning author Pearl S. Buck, is a beautiful book about one such parent's experiences. Ms. Buck eloquently describes the heartbreak and sorrow she experienced in raising a daughter who was mentally retarded as a result of a metabolic condition called PKU (phenylketonuria). But she also describes some of the 'benefits':

> [B]y this most sorrowful way I was compelled to tread, I learned respect and reverence for every human mind. It was my child who taught me to understand so clearly that all people are equal in their humanity and that all have the same human rights. None is to be considered less, as a human being, than any other, and each must be given his place and his safety in the world. I might never have learned this in any other way. I might have gone on in the arrogance of my own intolerance for those less able than myself. My child taught me humanity.[18]

How can we possibly determine the market value of such lessons? What tuition would we charge for learning humanity?

Despite these methodological flaws, it is clear that this 'bottom-line, cost-benefit analysis of human life' has become generally accepted in our society. Can anything be done to dispel this dark and sinister shadow of Mönchberg's smoke cloud?

Notes

1. Arthur Kent (1974) *The death doctors*, p. 256; Henry Friedlander (1995) *The origins of Nazi genocide: From euthanasia to the Final Solution*, pp. 92–93.
2. Robert J. Lifton (1986) *The Nazi doctors*, p. 52 (citing 'Secret Order', 18 August 1939, 'Re, duty to report malformed, etc. newborns').
3. For general descriptions of the establishment and operations of these 'killing centers', see ibid., pp. 45–79; Friedlander, op. cit.

4. 'Signs on the road leading to Hadamar warned that the danger of epidemics prohibited entry, but the chimney's smoke and the smell made local inhabitants aware of the nature of the operation.' Friedlander (1995), p. 93. 'The heavy smoke from the crematory building is said to be visible over Hadamar every day.' Lifton (1986), p. 75. '. . . [T]he citizens of Hadamar watch the smoke rise out of the chimney and are tortured with the ever-present thought of the poor sufferers, especially when the nauseating odours carried by the wind offend their nostrils.' Kent (1974), p. 256 (citing August 1941 letter from the Bishop of Limburg).

5. Kent (1974) p. 256 (citing August 1941 letter from the Bishop of Limburg).

6. This term is taken from the title of a book that was crucial to the development of Nazi Germany's killing programs, *Die Freigabe der Vernichtung lebensunwerten Leben* [The permission to destroy life unworthy of life], published in 1920 by a law professor named Karl Binding and a professor of psychiatry named Alfred Hoche. The authors stressed the burden such lives imposed on society, in comparison to their worth. Lifton (1986), pp. 46–47; Friedlander (1995), pp. 14–16.

7. Elizabeth Ring-Cassidy & Ian Gentles (2002) *Women's health after abortion: The medical and psychological evidence*, p. 158. For an insightful critique of the 'reassurance' rationale for prenatal testing, see Abby Lippman (1994) 'The genetic construction of testing' in Karen H. Rothenberg & Elizabeth J. Thompson (Eds.) *Women and prenatal testing: Facing the challenges of genetic technology*, p. 9.

8. Lippman argues that

> [W]hile a woman may have no control over or responsibility for the chromosomal occurrence of Down syndrome, she can control the birth of a child with this condition by being tested. Thus, if a child with Down syndrome is born to a woman who has refused testing, this becomes an event for which the child's mother is responsible because she could have prevented its occurrence. The individual is made into an agent of the state . . . Prenatal testing . . . reshapes the problem of disability so that it need not be ours collectively to solve (what will we do to embrace and accommodate those among us with disabilities?), but becomes . . . one for the individual woman to prevent (what will she do to avoid having a baby with a disability?) (Lippman, 1994, pp. 22–23).

9. *The Sunday Times*, July 4, 1999, as reported in *American Feminist* (Winter 1999–2000, p. 22). For similar arguments, see the sources cited in Anne Kerr & Tom Shakespeare (2002) *Genetic politics: From eugenics to genome*, p. 143.

10. Elena A. Gates, 'Prenatal genetic testing: Does it benefit pregnant women?', pp. 183, 189–190.

11. A chilling example of similar reasoning is found in a recent law review article proposing to deal with the costs of raising children with disabilities

by requiring all parents to pay a uniform per-child fee into a compulsory insurance plan. Parents who persist in bearing children with disabilities despite prenatal identification of the disability would be obligated to bear the cost of raising those children on their own, without assistance from the insurance fund. This article adopts the vocabulary, as well as the reasoning, of the Nazi eugenics programs; Part III of the article is entitled and directly addresses 'Lives Not Worth Living'. Erik Rakowski (2002) 'Who should pay for bad genes?', p. 1345.

12. Wrongful birth cases are brought by parents arguing that the birth of a child with a disability caused harm to them, by imposing on them the resultant burden of raising the child; wrongful life cases are brought by the person with a disability for damages resulting from being born with the disability. Legal causes of action for wrongful birth are recognized in 22 states; 3 states have rejected it. Kelly E. Rhinehart (2002a) 'The debate over wrongful birth and wrongful life', pp. 141, 142. Legal causes of action for wrongful life are recognized in only three states (California, Washington, and New Jersey), (Rhinehart. 2002b, p. 152). See also Jay Webber (2002) 'Better Off Dead?' p. 10.

13. James Meikle (2001) 'Down's children denied heart ops by biased doctors.'

14. Amy Dockser Marcus (2002) 'Ensuring your baby will be healthy: Embryo screening testing gains in popularity and controversy; Choosing a child's gender.' p. D1; Aaron Zitner (2002) 'A girl or boy, you pick', p. A1.

15. Garland E. Allan (2001) 'Is a new eugenics afoot?', p. 59.

16. One study calculated the lifetime cost to society of each child born with Down syndrome to be $451,000. Another calculated the cost to be at least $1 million. Tucker Carlson (1996) 'Eugenics American style: The abortion of Down syndrome babies', pp. 20, 22–23.

17. Zitner, op cit., quoting Deborah Kaplan, Executive Director of the World Institute on Disability in Oakland, California. See also Kerr & Shakespeare, pp. 143–145.

18. Pearl S. Buck (1992, 2nd ed.) *The child who never grew*, p. 78.

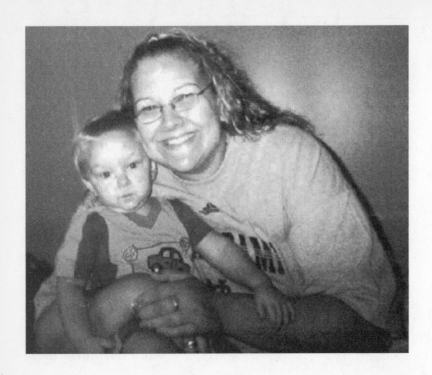

Stephanie Gillespie

Stephanie Gillespie is now a single mother of three: Paige, 7; Xander, 5; and Chandler, 3. She lives in Greensburg Indiana where she works for a company that provides services for adults with disabilities. Shortly after writing her contribution for *Defiant Birth*, she discovered she had cervical cancer. At the time of publication, it appears she has been successful in her battle against it.

Stephanie Gillespie

SO GLAD I LISTENED TO MY HEART

In September 2001 my whole world changed. Until that time, I thought I was invincible. In the perfect world I lived in, no harm could ever strike me. But then it all changed. The walls crumbled and the earth turned to ashes.

The first blow was the terrorist strike on 9-11. Those horrible men struck a chord of pain that resonated in my heart. This pain was accompanied by the fear that maybe everything would not always be all right. I had believed that no matter what happened, my family could always protect me. But now, with planes crashing into cities like bolts of lightning from an angry god, I began to question the security that I had held so dear.

In the weeks that followed the attacks, I began to feel strange. I was sick in the mornings and tired at night. At first I thought it was some physical manifestation of the pain in my heart. But I soon recognised the symptoms. My suspicions were confirmed when my doctor told me I was pregnant. Although this was the fourth life that had sparked inside me, it somehow felt different. With my previous children, when I learned I was pregnant, I was overwhelmed with joy. However, this time I felt no elation. My husband and I were struck with disbelief. We had taken precautions to prevent this very thing.

The early months were less than happy. My husband, the primary provider for our family, lost his job. To remain afloat in the downward spiral of the recession, his company had to downsize. He had not been there for long, so I guess they saw him as expendable. We had to survive on my income. My son, who was 2 at the time, had been having problems. I work with the developmentally disabled and recognised some of the signs. After subjecting him to a battery of tests, he was diagnosed with a seizure disorder. With my husband losing his job, we also lost our medical insurance. Because of my son's disorder, his mental development was delayed. We had to take him to specialists in child neurology and to psychologists. With the expenses piling up, we found ourselves in a situation we had never been in before. We were finally connected with state funded agencies to assist us in finding insurance for the children and my pregnancy.

After enduring this struggle for three months, it was time for my check-up and ultrasound. I had been so anxious to see my unborn. I thought that watching the life on the monitor would be just what I needed to lift my spirits and restore my hope in the future. We had no reason to think anything was wrong.

My husband was starting a new job that day – he went to work and I went to the appointment. The technician entered the room. It was the same woman who had done the ultrasounds for my two other children. She was a cheerful lady and I looked forward to seeing her expressions as she discovered the different areas of my baby and pointed them out to me. I remember thinking how she must have the most wonderful job in the world. She began as she had done in the past, by pouring the gel on my belly while saying how sorry she was that no one had yet invented a warmer for the gel. After this ritual, she began to probe my abdomen in search of my child. She had a very difficult time finding anything. I was concerned, but she told me not to worry; the doctor had probably got the due date wrong. When I returned two weeks later, I was anxious to see how much my child had grown. I had always been fascinated with how much my children developed, and used their growth as a convenient excuse to treat myself to some ice-cream or chocolate. No matter what they say, I am convinced that a chocolate-chip cookie-dough blizzard from Dairy Queen is the absolute best thing a woman can eat for her developing baby!

After taking some measurements, the technician told me that my baby's new due date was closer to the end of June than early June. I was telling her my birthday was 15 June, when her expression soured. She told me to wait, she would be right back. My stomach rose into my throat. My heart began to beat ferociously. What had she found? What was going on? My thoughts raced at a thunderous pace. It seemed like hours before she returned. When she did, the doctor was following her. She pointed at the screen and they spoke in low tones. He nodded. Seeing the confused grimace on my face, the technician explained that the amniotic fluid was very low and that the baby was very small. It also appeared my child was a good candidate for Down syndrome. It looked like my child's stomach was outside his body and there was a hole in his intestinal wall. The doctor referred me to the Indiana University Medical Center in Indianapolis. As I left the office, tears began to pour down my cheeks. I cried the entire drive home and through the rest of the day. I had miscarried my last child and the emotions of that time came rushing back.

One week later I was at the medical center where I was put through a raft of tests. In addition to the earlier diagnosis, the doctors added the possibility of toxoplasmosis and water on the brain. I just sat there, heart broken. I do not even remember what they said. I had miscarried my daughter and now I was going to lose my son. (Due to the genetic testing and prior ultrasounds we knew the baby was a boy.) Even if I didn't lose him, how could I take care of him? I already had a child at home who took much of our energy, dealing with his disabilities.

I made my way down the hall to the genetic counsellor. I was not ready for this, I wanted to run away and hide from the pain.

The counsellor explained the tests and the conclusion the doctors had come to. They recommended an abortion. She told me that my child's prospects of even being born alive were slim and that if he were born, he would have no quality of life. She also told me that there really were no alternatives. She turned to retrieve her appointment book from her desk. She looked back at me and told me that by having an abortion I was doing the right thing, and before I knew it I would be pregnant again and have a healthy baby. She opened the book to schedule the abortion. I was bewildered. She asked if I had any questions. I asked why we would even consider abortion when all we had heard up to this point was that the baby may have a defect, or may not make it through the pregnancy. How could I even consider aborting my child based on a theory? She suggested an amniocentesis test to screen for genetic disorders. She told me this would remove any doubts that I was doing the right thing with an abortion. I asked why this would not be performed before even recommending an abortion. She told me that in cases such as mine there is little doubt as to the outcome, so it is unnecessary, but they would do it if it eased my mind. I returned for the procedure. In addition to the amniocentesis I was scheduled to see a paediatric cardiologist. I went in thinking that there was nothing they could do to make me change my mind about the abortion.

The amniocentesis proceeded painfully. The results would take a few weeks. I was then sent to the cardiologist. She said my baby's heart could not be seen very well. She found a hole in his heart that should close up by the time he was born, but she couldn't tell us that for sure. She didn't tell us anything that was certain except that he had a heart. We knew nothing more than when we first went in. We were offered information on the abortion process once again. We left.

The much-awaited phone call came from the genetic counsellor.

I remember the sound of her voice distinctly – it was monotone and lifeless. She told me the tests had come back negative. She informed me there were strands of genetic defects that are undetectable and just because the test came back in our favour there still had to be a problem with my child. I was instructed to come back in a month for more testing. I once again questioned why it was necessary to continue testing. She said that since we were choosing to continue the pregnancy, we should give the doctors a head start on the problems that my child may face.

I felt very strong going into the appointment. I had stayed true to my heart and to my child and so far everything came back in our favour. I couldn't imagine what else they could possibly say to diminish my confidence. The doctors ordered another ultrasound to chart the growth of the baby in the last month. The technician left to retrieve the doctors and share the findings. They now had a new diagnosis – this time it was dwarfism. I almost laughed out loud. Perhaps they needed something to hold onto so they didn't look so stupid for pushing me to have an abortion? They requested I come back every month until delivery. Then they would set up a caesarean section. I suggested that due to the findings being less than life threatening I should continue to be monitored by my regular obstetrician. The doctors relented, and when I stepped out the door I never looked back.

Going back to my regular obstetrician was like returning home from a long trip. I had one final ultrasound and he came in to observe. The hunt was on once again. The doctor and the technician spoke softly at the end of the table. The doctor questioned the size of my last baby. My son had weighed nearly ten pounds and we were expecting close to the same for our next child. He told me that at this point my son was lucky to be weighing four to five pounds; he was not growing as well as he should be. His lungs needed more time to develop; if he were born now, more than likely, he would not survive on his own. I cried all the way home. I felt so helpless, so responsible for his struggle. Something was wrong, but no one could tell me what it was.

I was scheduled for an induction on 23 June. I arrived at the hospital at 7 pm. I hated leaving my other two children with their grandparents, but they were looking forward to it. My daughter referred to it as a vacation. That made it a little bit easier. It was an eventless night. I was dilated to 3 cm as I fell asleep. I woke up to the nurse explaining to my husband that they were going to begin a petocin drip to get my labour started. This was done at 7 am and my labour went on for hours. At 2 pm I received an epidural. This stopped my pain, but also stopped my labour. The baby's heart rate started to dip, setting off frequent alarms. My blood pressure was steadily rising. The doctor was coming in and out every ten minutes or so. He would ask how I was feeling and tell me he didn't like where this was going. I began to get very scared. I thought to myself – the only reason the baby is having such a hard time is because something is terribly wrong with him. I was afraid he was dying.

The clock moved slowly, but I listened to every tick. I tried not to cry and not to imagine the worst. It was 11:50 pm and the alarm had just gone off again. The door to my room flew open and in came a string of nurses and the doctor. Wires were unplugged and my husband was fitted with surgery attire. Everyone was rushing around. I was being transferred to the operating room down the hall. The doctor told me if he did not deliver the baby now, he wasn't going to make it. He said he could deliver the baby in 30 seconds and he thought it would come down to that. This sent me into an extreme state of panic. I thought of everything we had been through. My son might die. He was already a huge part of my life. I grabbed the nurse and begged her that no matter what the outcome, I wanted to see him. I made her promise that I could hold him and touch him. I needed to tell him that I loved him. She looked at me sympathetically and told me she would get him to me as soon as she could.

On 25 June 2002, at 12:03 am, I heard a cry that rejuvenated my soul. My son was born: 5 lb 12 oz, 19 inches! He was screaming so loud – like a declaration of his achievement, his life. My son was here and I could see him and touch him and listen to him breathe. I was exhausted. My husband followed him to the nursery while I went to the recovery room. About 7 hours later I got to hold my son, Chandler, for the first time. I was so overwhelmed with excitement that I didn't notice the oddity of the paediatrician bringing him to me. She just smiled and asked how I was doing. I told her that everything was fine now, but her face told another story. Chandler was going to be taken for a CAT scan. She showed me that his head was swollen. His soft spot was enormous – she laid almost two fingers into it. She said she had never seen a soft spot so huge and feared he might have water on the brain. She also told me that if that was not the case, she was concerned about the possibility of permanent brain damage, or mental retardation.

I asked my husband to leave me alone with Chandler for a little while before the X-ray technician came in. I didn't know what to think. I held this sleeping angel and tried to imagine what kind of life he might have. I pulled him close to my chest and cried until I couldn't cry anymore. We had been through so much. I couldn't give up now. I had never understood the depth a mother could love her child until that moment. I thought of my other children at home and the hardship that would face us, but I didn't care. At 2 pm my phone rang. I was alone with Chandler, enjoying our solitude. The call was from the paediatrician. The CAT scan came back fine. She said that we would have to wait and see how he developed to determine if there were any developmental issues. I was so relieved.

We left the hospital a few days later to start our lives as a family. Chandler is now eighteen months old. He has not only met his developmental goals, he has exceeded them. My child has no signs of any of the disabilities that were predicted for him. If I had chosen to abort him, I would have destroyed a perfectly healthy baby. Every life is special and everyone has a purpose. I am very glad I listened to my heart and not the doctors. When he comes running out of the living room when I come home to give me slobbery kisses and wrap his little arms around me so tight, I know I did the right thing.

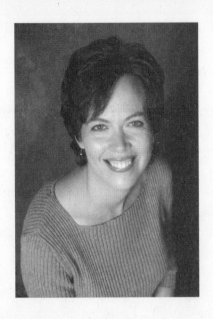

Amy Kuebelbeck

Amy Kuebelbeck is a former journalist and author of *Waiting with Gabriel: A story of cherishing a baby's brief life* (also published in Italy as *Aspettando Gabriel*). She lives with her husband and their two daughters in Saint Paul, Minnesota USA. Amy is an avid musician who plays piano, acoustic and classical guitar. She began guitar lessons when she was 7 and thanks her parents for not allowing her to quit to join Girl Scouts instead.

Amy Kuebelbeck

GABRIEL WAS GOING TO DIE,
BUT FIRST HE WAS GOING TO LIVE

'You have a beautiful baby,' the ultrasound technician said quietly. She was studying the flickering images on her screen, staring intently at the shadows of the tiny heart. I think she had already seen that our baby was going to die.

What followed was an extraordinary journey of grief, joy and love as we waited with Gabriel, simultaneously preparing for our son's birth and for his death. Despite some wrenchingly aggressive surgical options, no one could give our son a good heart. So we set out to give him a good life, even if it was going to be short.

As Gabriel grew and settled into position for birth, I could almost always feel one of his little feet just to the right of my navel. No matter where I went, I could take him with me. And when the grief came crashing over me, I could seek solace in curling around him. Among all the people being affected by Gabriel's expected death, I began to feel like the fortunate one, because he was so close to me.

The months of waiting culminated in two-and-a-half hours of cradling Gabriel in our arms, in the same bed where he was born, surrounded by family and friends until his imperfect little heart finally stopped beating altogether.

People sometimes are astonished – and perhaps a little horrified – that I walked around pregnant for three-and-a-half months carrying a baby I knew would die. We were well aware that aborting Gabriel was an option and, in some circles, an expectation.

Now that we've been through it, I believe that aborting my pregnancy would have been disastrous on many levels. Most important, it would have cut Gabriel's natural life short for no good reason.

It would not have been a shortcut through our grief. If anything, our grief would have been magnified. We would have been left with only the raw pain and without the memories of our son and the time-tested rituals of grief to soften it. Perhaps some people thought we were bringing grief upon ourselves by continuing the pregnancy and having a full funeral and burial. Some must have thought that we should just get on with our lives. But for that brief time, Gabriel was our life. Other than caring for our two daughters, there was nothing more important in our lives than waiting with Gabriel, giving him the full measure of our time and attention and love.

I also felt that ending the pregnancy early would have contributed to the perception that the loss of an unborn baby is of little consequence. And we would still have been in shock a week or two later, when others would have been expecting us to get over it already. Instead, my growing belly was a constant reminder to others of what we were going through. Perhaps that meant that everywhere we went, death was an uninvited and unwelcome guest. But it also resulted in our receiving an extraordinary level of support, rare for parents grieving the loss of their 'invisible' baby.

Aborting the pregnancy would have meant denying ourselves the life-changing, bittersweet, exquisite experience of holding our beautiful full-term son and hearing his cries. We didn't realise until later how crucial and sustaining those memories would be. Ending the pregnancy early would have meant rejecting a gift.

I believe that ending our pregnancy early would have caused us real emotional harm, as well as closed us off from the extraordinary gifts that we and our families and close friends were able to experience as we all waited with Gabriel.

Yes, Gabriel was going to die. But first he was going to live.

Support for continuing a pregnancy: Perinatal hospice

As prenatal testing becomes increasingly routine, more parents are learning devastating news before their babies are born. In too many places, the ability to diagnose has raced ahead of the ability to care for these families and their babies. But in a beautiful and practical response, a few hospitals around the US are starting perinatal hospice programs for families who wish to continue their pregnancies with babies who likely will die before, during, or after birth.

Under the conventional hospice model, services do not begin until the baby is born or is discharged from the hospital, which is of little help when a baby has a life expectancy of hours or even minutes. Perinatal hospices, in contrast, are intended to support families from the time of diagnosis, when their grief journey begins. In the words of one perinatal hospice program, Deeya, based at Children's Hospitals and Clinics in Minneapolis: 'We walk with families through pregnancy, birth, life, and bereavement – supporting the dignity and value of each life.' It's a tender, life-affirming response to one of the most heartbreaking challenges of prenatal testing.

In a 2001 article in the *American Journal of Obstetrics and Gynecology*, Dr Byron C. Calhoun and Dr Nathan J. Hoeldtke proposed a perinatal hospice model that incorporates perinatal grief management and hospice care. They recommended using a multidisciplinary team approach – including anesthesia service, labor and delivery nurses, social workers and chaplains – to care for the family before, during, and after birth.

In the US, perinatal hospice service is now offered through San Diego Hospice and Palliative Care; Cincinnati Children's Hospital Medical Center; Kansas City Hospice; Angel Babies of Hinds Hospice, Fresno, California; and others.

Even in areas without a formal program, caregivers can offer services in the spirit of hospice. During the remainder of the pregnancy, for example, caregivers can provide frequent ultrasound pictures for the parents to keep, help draw up specialised birth plans, talk with parents about ideas for creating memories, and help plan for baptism or a blessing if parents wish. Caregivers can discuss difficult but practical matters of decisions about medical intervention after birth, organ donation, burial or other disposition of the body, and how to cope when the mother's milk supply comes in. Once the baby arrives, caregivers can help families keep the baby comfortable (if the baby is still alive), take photographs, collect handprints and footprints and locks of hair, bathe the baby, perhaps rock the baby and sing or read to him or her, and invite family members and close friends to see the baby and enter into the bittersweet circle.

Elisabeth Kübler-Ross once said, 'Parents are often not given permission by family or friends to mourn the death of their baby, and they are very often left alone in an apparently unsympathetic world, not knowing how to feel and not knowing how to cope.' Thanks to the efforts of bereaved parents and groups such as SANDS (Stillbirth and Neonatal Death Society) Australia, SHARE Pregnancy and Infant Loss Support and others, hospital practices and societal attitudes regarding miscarriage, stillbirth and neonatal death are gradually changing. Perinatal hospice service builds upon these efforts.

Caregivers who may view continuing a pregnancy following a lethal prenatal diagnosis as an exercise in futility or denial may wish to reconsider their assumptions. Many families see it as an effort to honor their child and to embrace whatever time they may be able to have together, even if it is only before birth.

'Parental responses have been overwhelmingly positive,' Dr Calhoun and Dr Hoeldtke report. 'These parents are allowed the bitter-sweetness of their child's birth and too-soon departure. Grief lessens as time passes and parents rest secure in the knowledge that they shared in their baby's life and treated the child with the same dignity as a terminally ill adult.'

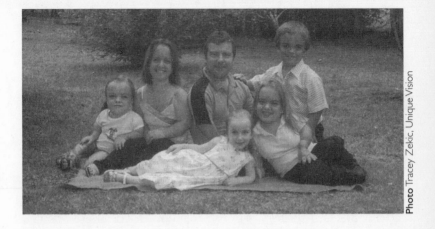

Photo Tracey Zekic, Unique Vision

Leisa Whitaker

Leisa Whitaker shares a house with her husband James and their four children: Sarah, 18; Chloe, 15; Tim, 14; and Georgia, 9; along with a menagerie of pets including two dogs, a cat, two budgies, two rabbits, four guinea pigs and tropical and coldwater fish. Leisa enjoys quilting and stitcheries and has developed an unfortunate habit of starting new quilts before finishing the previous one. She loves reading and writing and hopes to complete a course in Professional Writing and Editing in the near future.

Leisa Whitaker

I WOULDN'T SWAP THEM FOR ANYTHING

I was born with achondroplasia, the most common form of dwarfism. A baby with achondroplasia is born once in every 26,000 births and occurs as a chance mutation in a gene. There is usually no family history of dwarfism; in other words, most people with achondroplasia have parents who are average-sized. That's how it was in my case. I am the eldest of seven children, and the only one with this condition. My family were wonderful. To them I was just me. I was loved, nurtured, disciplined and treated just the same as anyone else. I was a strong, healthy, active child. I had ballet lessons, climbed trees, rode my bike, swam, camped and hiked with my family and was surrounded by friends. My child-hood was free of any extra problems that can be associated with achondroplasia. This experience later formed the basis of my decision to have children.

For as long as I can remember I wanted to be a mother. I had dolls that I would nurture as though they were real. My mother recalls that while she was feeding one of her babies, I would get one of my own, sit right alongside her and 'breastfeed' as well. I loved it when my mother had babies. I wanted to help out in any way I could. I was the eldest in a large family so there was always a baby around to cuddle and love.

I met my husband James during my early teens at a camp for short-statured teenagers held by the Short Statured People of Australia – a support group for people with dwarfism and their families. My family had been members since I was 6 years old but this was the first event that I had really participated in. Over the course of a number of years, James and I became close friends and fell in love. It was a long-distance relationship as I lived in the suburbs of Melbourne and he was up on the mid-north coast of New South Wales. We saw each other as often as we could.

When I discovered I was pregnant during mid-1986, it was a very traumatic time. I was halfway through my Diploma of Teaching, and all I wanted to do was leave university and move to Port Macquarie to be with James and his family. At the time, I left university without much thought, as I simply panicked and felt I would not be able to cope with having a baby and studying as well. Now that I am older I wish I'd had the maturity to finish off my second year at university and defer the final year until after the baby was born, as I had plenty of support from family and friends to make this happen. Initially we did move to Port Macquarie but I became very homesick and missed the support of my parents. We also realised that living in Port Macquarie and being under the care of the doctors in Sydney was going to be very difficult to manage, so we decided we would move back down to Melbourne. My family were very supportive of us and welcomed James into the family.

The thought that we could have other more serious issues to consider did not enter our heads. James was born with pseudoachondroplasia – a dwarfing condition that doesn't really become physically apparent until the age of eighteen months. It is similar to achondroplasia in that it causes restricted growth in the arms and legs but also causes problems in the joints, particularly the hips, knees and ankles. Unlike achondroplasia, the facial features are not affected. Both James and I had been strong, healthy children, free of surgery and other medical intervention. We had no reason to suspect that any children we had wouldn't have the same experiences and assumed that all would be well.

It wasn't until a visit to the genetics specialist in Sydney was scheduled that we learned the facts. I remember sitting in his rooms listening as he explained that there was a 25 percent chance that our child could still inherit the dominant achondroplasia gene and the dominant pseudoachondroplasia gene – a combination that they had never seen before anywhere in the world. They had no idea of what effect this would have on the baby – whether it would die soon after birth or if it would have lasting physical problems. They had absolutely nothing to go on. Having told us this, the specialist offered us an abortion. He asked us to think about whether we wanted to bring another dwarf baby into the world. It was something I hadn't even thought of. This was our child! Why would we not want her? Why would the world not accept our child?

I remember sitting on that chair in the doctor's rooms. I hugged my knees to my chest in a protective gesture and said inside myself, 'Don't worry, little baby. Nobody's going to hurt you.' I would have only been about ten weeks pregnant at the time, but already our baby was real, alive and growing. I could feel her in my soul.

To give them their dues, not all the specialists were the same. After we decided that we would move back to Melbourne to be closer to my family, we went to visit the genetics specialists at the Royal Children's Hospital. Although they gave us the same factual information, they were a lot more supportive of our decisions, and painted a brighter picture of our child's future. We knew that because of the size of my pelvis, there was no way I would be able to give birth naturally, and a caesarean was my only option. I was placed under the care of the obstetricians at the Queen Victoria Medical Centre who were more practised in dealing with 'difficult' cases such as mine.

There were people who questioned our rights to continue the pregnancy and have our baby. One extended family member expressed that if I was her daughter, I would have been marched off straight away to the abortion clinic to have the pregnancy terminated. There was talk all around us that we never actually heard directly, but we knew it was going on, and it hurt just the same. The mother of one of my best friends is, to this day, still horrified that I could have even considered having children knowing that I could pass on the achondroplasia gene, even if I had married and had children with an average-sized man. Another acquaintance has said that she feels extreme pity for our children. All of this talk has had an impact on me over the years – not that it has deterred me in any way, but it has illustrated that even though people may treat you normally and relate to you as they would any other person, deep down you are still 'different' and somehow have to live by different rules. I wonder if they even comprehend the idea that a person living with a physical difference such as mine is capable of normal feelings such as love, physical desire and a strong maternal instinct. Maybe that's what challenges them.

Whenever I went for an antenatal check-up, there were always students wanting to learn about my condition, my pregnancy and me. At the time I didn't question anything that happened, as it was a whole new experience to both James and myself, and both of us were overwhelmed by everything. The students were always very polite and sensitive, but it got tiresome answering the same questions over and over. I had numerous ultrasounds that mapped the growth of the baby. It wasn't until about week 28 that it showed a small variation. The head circumference was slightly larger than it should have been, although the doctor said that it was still well within the range of 'normal', and they could not ascertain if the baby had any type of dwarfism. This didn't perturb us at all.

I had another ultrasound at about 33 weeks. We saw a profile of our baby on the screen and even James and I could tell that she had achondroplasia. The doctor doing the ultrasound said to us,

'This baby looks like you, Leisa!' At this point we did not know the sex of our baby; all we knew was that we were having a baby that was going to be a dwarf, and because of the lives that we had had so far, that was fine by us.

I was put into hospital about ten days before my caesarean was scheduled, so that they could keep an eye on me and make sure I didn't go into early labour. Their fears were unfounded and on 18 March 1987, at 10:29 am, under the watchful eye of her father, Sarah Amy Whitaker entered the world feet first. She was floppy and it took her a while to get going, so she was taken to the Special Care Nursery to be monitored.

After my caesarean I woke to a searing agony that told me I had, indeed, had an operation. There was a feeling of emptiness too. When you have a caesarean under general anaesthetic you are wheeled into the operating theatre pregnant, and when you wake up you're not. It's all taken out of your hands and is done for you. With a natural delivery I see the mother as an active participant who gets to witness her baby coming into the world. When I woke up I just knew that my baby was no longer there and was being cared for in another part of the hospital.

I kept insisting that I wanted to see my baby. I wouldn't rest until I had seen her, despite the fact that I had just had surgery no more than three hours earlier and the nursing staff wanted me to rest. They got me a wheelchair and wheeled me to the Special Care Nursery.

And there she was.

'Wow. She's got a big head.'

That was my first recognisable thought.

Her daddy was holding her, giving her a bottle. He looked so young – almost a boy himself, but there was no missing that unmistakable look of pride and awe in his face. It is seared into my memory forever.

They placed her in my arms.

Congratulations.

'Hello, little baby.' All I felt was curiosity. She was wrapped tightly in her blanket. Caesar babies find it difficult to maintain their body heat, but I didn't know that. I just started unwrapping her. I needed to see her. It was like I just needed to confirm that this was a baby – a real live baby, and that she was mine. She certainly didn't feel like mine, but I knew that she was.

I don't know when it happened. I can't even remember the next time I saw her, but some time over the next couple of days I fell totally in love with her. I realised I was changed forever and would never be the same person again. Nobody told me that our souls would knit together so completely, that I would be just so totally sold out to this little life. It is such a powerful thing and I am still in awe of it eighteen years later.

It was difficult, having Sarah in the Special Care Nursery. I had no idea what was being done to her and who was looking after her. Often things were done without my knowledge or consent. I have a vague recollection of doctors telling me they had given her a cranial ultrasound to check for hydrocephalus, but they did that as I was still recovering from the general anaesthetic, which wasn't the most ideal time to ask my permission for anything. Sarah was a floppy baby and very sleepy, which meant she had feeding problems. I was very keen to breastfeed and had an ample supply, but she was reluctant to feed and started to lose weight quite rapidly. To top it all off, doctors would come on their rounds with an entourage of students, take her out of her cot, undress her and examine her without my consent. Once I was at the end of a feed and the entourage came around and actually asked me if they could examine Sarah after I had finished feeding her. I answered in the negative, explaining that she was sleepy and we were having feeding problems. The doctor said to me, 'Well, the students have to learn!' which meant that they were going to do it regardless of my wishes. I was extremely upset and left the nursery in tears. Later on I spoke to the nursing unit manager and asked that there be no more students examining my baby; a note was put on her cot stating my wishes. I don't know if they honoured my request, but I have a feeling they didn't.

I was left with the feeling of being powerless and having no rights, both as a person and a mother. I learned a lot from this experience, and with my subsequent pregnancies we were very vocal and forthright when it came to what we would allow and what we wouldn't. I do agree that student doctors need to learn from different patients, but I am totally against the way they disregarded our rights to privacy. Since then we have surrounded ourselves with professionals who know us, and we don't feel guilty if we say no to students or any medical photographic documentation we feel isn't necessary.

Sarah was the joy of our lives. After the feeding problems were resolved we settled into our new family life. Sarah progressed well, although she had a lumbar kyphosis – a curve in the lower part of her spine – that needed monitoring closely. As far as we knew she only had achondroplasia like me.

When Sarah was two we decided we'd try for another baby. She was doing well, although her spine was causing a few concerns. Sarah learned to walk when she was about two-and-a-half years old, which is not unusual for a child with achondroplasia, and she was healthy. We were overjoyed when I discovered I was pregnant again. This time I took matters into my own hands. I said I wasn't going to have any students come and see me, nor was there to be any student come and poke and prod my baby. I only had two ultrasounds – the standard 16-week ultrasound to check that all is well and the dates are correct, and a final ultrasound at about 32 weeks, where we discovered that this baby too was going to have achondroplasia. Our precious Chloe Hannah was born in March 1990.

It wasn't long after Chloe's birth that we were at a regular genetics clinic visit and our specialist looked at Sarah and said, 'You know, I believe Sarah has pseudoachondroplasia as well.' It was a diagnosis that didn't really shock us at the time. In fact, it helped to explain why Sarah had floppier joints than other children her age with achondroplasia. They termed her a 'compound heterozygote', in other words, she had both the dominant achon-droplasia gene and the dominant pseudoachondroplasia gene. Looking back on it all now, I know I didn't really fully understand what impact this diagnosis was going to have on Sarah, and later on Chloe. Chloe was diagnosed as having both conditions a lot earlier than Sarah, as by then we all knew what we were looking for.

We had four children. Our son, Timothy Jordan, was born in 1991 and, thankfully, he was diagnosed with simple achondroplasia on the day that Chloe was diagnosed with both. Georgia Kate arrived in May 1996. I had avoided the genetics clinic during my pregnancy with Georgia, as I didn't want to see the concern on their faces and become worried myself. During the final ultra-sound, the baby looked unaffected by dwarfism. We were overjoyed. In the back of our minds we knew it was possible that she could have pseudoachondroplasia, but at least we knew that she was not going to have both.

After Tim's birth, the doctors recommended that I didn't have any more children, as the caesareans were becoming increasingly difficult. With Tim it took quite a while for them to cut through all the scar tissue, which of course meant the anaesthetic was affecting the baby for a longer period of time. This played on my mind a lot while I was pregnant with Georgia. The surgery was very difficult and the anaesthetic had affected her to the point where she required a narcotic antagonist to reverse the effects that my general anaesthetic had on her after she was delivered. We decided she would be our last.

Georgia was diagnosed with pseudoachondroplasia at nine months of age. I had reached a stage where I was so hopeful that she was average-sized I knew I needed to know once and for all. I know a lot of people have questioned why I felt that way. Why wouldn't I? I am just like every other mother, hoping for the best for all her children. I accepted whatever came our way, but I never wished for any of them to have dwarfism. We would not have thought Georgia the 'odd one out' if she had been average-sized, no more than I was the 'odd one out' being the only one with dwarfism in my average-sized family. She would have just been our Georgia.

Georgia was X-rayed and after the results were reported our specialists informed us that she did have pseudoachondroplasia. Actually, I could tell as soon as the doctors walked into the room. There was just something in their faces that told me all I needed to know. They handled the situation with compassion and kindness, not assuming anything. I am very grateful for that, as I was very upset at the time and mourned for a couple of days. It was an experience that taught me compassion for other parents who have had a child diagnosed with a medical condition. We at least were almost expecting this diagnosis. Usually, this happens so out of the blue that it comes as a shock and may take a very long time to come to terms with, before the parents can move on.

Sarah and Chloe have limited mobility now. They are able to walk around our home, but use powered wheelchairs when out and about and at school. Having both conditions affects them in different ways. Both have very weak wrists and fingers but are very strong in the shoulders and upper arm. They have weaker legs, which means that walking long distances is a struggle. Their spinal curvature requires monitoring every six months. Things that other teenagers take for granted – even putting on socks and tying shoes – take longer for both girls, but the sense of achievement they get when gaining a little more physical independence is priceless! Both girls are only one metre tall, however this is within the average height range for people with pseudoachondroplasia.

I am so in love with my children. They are amazing. Sarah is a vibrant young woman, devoted to her friends, and has a special affinity with young children. Chloe is a quiet girl with a very dry sense of humour. She loves to sing and is passionate about animals. Tim is a thoughtful young man who is so caring towards his sisters. From a very young age, and without being told, he has been aware of Sarah and Chloe's limitations and has adapted accordingly. Tim opens doors for them, moves stools around for them and generally helps out whenever he is needed without a word of complaint. When he learned to walk at twenty months, even though he was the youngest at the time, he was the one who had to walk next to the pram or stroller, as it was Sarah and Chloe who still needed it. Georgia is so sweet and caring to others. She loves to dance and sing and wants a life on the stage. All of them touch the hearts of anyone they come in contact with. They are intelligent, thoughtful, polite and a joy to be around. They don't want to be pitied for all the things they may not be able to do. They want to be celebrated for the people they are!

Yes, we have had problems. Each one of the children has undergone some sort of surgery. It is during these times that I falter and become not so 'defiant'. We also live in a society that worships physical perfection and doesn't seem to tolerate anyone or anything that does not conform to what is normal and acceptable. It seems to be harder and harder to step out of our front door and face the world, as it's a world that doesn't tolerate difference. Yes, we have every opportunity open to us. People with dwarfism can become doctors, lawyers, schoolteachers, architects, tradespeople and so on, thanks to the laws that uphold equality of opportunity and anti-discrimination. However with prenatal diagnosis becoming so routine, the human race is now able to choose who is acceptable and who is not. Seeing people like us flies in the face of 'perfection', and I think society finds us a challenge to deal with, as we are normal, intelligent human beings living in a body that is not viewed as acceptable. I was devastated when I heard about the case involving the late-term abortion (at 32 weeks) of a baby that had been diagnosed as having achondroplasia. For a long while I had thought that we were 'safe' because achondroplasia would not normally be a condition a doctor would be looking for and by the time it was obvious it would be too 'late' to 'do something about it'. And what did aborting that baby say about us? Did society think we were better off dead? I felt so upset for the mother of that child, wondering why she was in a place where she felt that there was no hope for that baby, or was it just a case of a world so obsessed with physical perfection that she was made to feel bad for producing someone who didn't fit into that mould?

I find myself wondering about the image I portray to the world. How does the world see me? I evaluate my day sometimes. What am I doing that is so different to other thirty-something women who are working mothers? What aspect about my life is so terrible that that poor woman felt that she had no other option but to abort her baby? Was there something I could have done to show her that life for that baby would have been okay – different than she expected, but okay?

I could never have prepared myself for what being a mother is. I have found it to be the most wonderful, amazing, awe-inspiring, terrifying, heartbreaking, joyful, rollercoaster ride in life that anyone could possibly experience. I know that I was meant to fulfil my desire to be a mother, regardless of the many genetic, ethical, moral arguments that I have had from others and even in my own head sometimes. I do have feelings of guilt from time to time, but when I look at these four wonderful people who love life and have the capacity to contribute to the world in many different and special ways, I know they were meant to be here. Who knows what they will achieve in their lifetime? Who knows how many people they will reach out to, touch and inspire? Having these children has also given me a glimpse into the lives of other families we meet at the clinics in the hospital – other families who are facing the future with courage and perseverance in situations even more challenging than ours. They encourage and inspire me.

There is no going back. And I don't want to – even in the worst, dark times where I feel as though I am losing my mind with all the fear and worry. Even though we are facing a future that is unknown, we now have four precious pieces of immortality – 'with their father's good looks and my sense of style' (in the words of Julia Roberts in *Steel Magnolias*). We get to spend an eternity with them. I wouldn't swap that for anything.

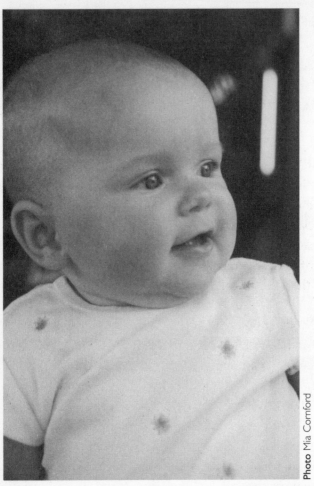

Photo Mia Cornford

Alison Streeter

Alison Streeter lives in Sydney, Australia, with her husband Mark and daughters, Emily and Amelia. She feels a strong sense of responsibility to speak up for those who can't speak for themselves. She also really enjoys spending time with her family and friends.

Alison Streeter

THIS BABY WOULD BE LOVED

'I'm pregnant!' I scream as we study the home test results together. We are so excited and thankful. We tell our family and friends the wonderful news at nine weeks. Joy!

How quickly things can change. What follows took place between weeks ten and twelve of my pregnancy. The experiences that I went through are embedded in my mind and the emotions that I felt at the time are still raw.

A dear friend and her small child come for lunch. We have a lovely time as we chat and watch our children play together. After a few hours, I notice and point out a rash on her child's back. We think nothing of it.

A phone call the following day. 'Ali, I've just taken Sam to the doctor and he's got German measles. I thought I should let you know. I'm sorry.'

I do my best to sound calm on the phone, not wanting to cause my friend any more distress, but once I'm off the phone I feel ill and faint. What she doesn't know is that my body is resistant to the rubella vaccine. I wait until my husband gets home to tell him. I spend the evening researching the implications of contracting German measles whilst pregnant.

I visit my GP the next morning and discover that the incubation period for German measles is two weeks. This means a number of things:

1. one blood test today and another in two weeks to see if I actually

do contract German measles;

2. two weeks of agonising while waiting;
3. total isolation for two weeks from the rest of the community so that I don't infect anyone else;
4. a phone call to my obstetrician;
5. lots of prayer.

The obstetrician recommended I have an ultrasound and see a genetic counsellor tomorrow. He also recommended that I attend a particular ultrasound clinic. Off I go.

I arrive at the clinic and am immediately sent to an isolation room so that I don't come into contact with anyone else. A few minutes later I have an ultrasound that confirms that I am ten weeks pregnant. The midwife gingerly asks me if I understand the implications of contracting German measles. I tell her I've read a little. I then ask to get a photo of my baby printed. She looks at me strangely and I say to her, 'Whatever the outcome, I'm not going to pretend that this baby wasn't conceived.' She smiles an understanding smile and gives me my first photo of my baby. Then it's back into the isolation room.

This is where things get quite ugly. I wait a few minutes and embrace the opportunity to gaze lovingly at the picture of my beautiful baby. In comes the genetic counsellor. She is young and confident. She hands me a wad of paper and says, 'Read these and I'll be back soon to talk.' The documents were downloaded from medical websites and were all on congenital rubella syndrome [CRS]. It took about 5 minutes to read the distressing documents. Through these articles I discovered that the worst time to come into contact with German measles is in week ten of pregnancy – lucky me! – and that although the consequences of CRS are varied, the worst case scenario is having a baby who is born blind, deaf, brain damaged, whose bones won't calcify properly and who has lesions on their internal organs. I read and re-read this material several times.

After 20 minutes of waiting for the genetic counsellor to return, I phone my husband. I'm in a state of deep shock and highly stressed. The isolation isn't helping.

After 30 minutes of sitting holding a photo of my baby in one hand and these terrible medical documents in the other, I feel as though I can't cope any longer. The genetic counsellor still hasn't arrived. I fall asleep – the only strategy I have left.

After I had been waiting for 40 minutes, the genetic counsellor finally arrives and ushers me to her office.

The ugliness gets uglier . . .

GC: It's a shame that the ultrasound confirms that you are ten weeks pregnant.

Me: Oh well, there's nothing we can do about it.

GC: Do you understand how serious CRS is?

Me: Yes.

GC: Do you understand how serious it is to contract German measles in the tenth week of pregnancy?

Me: I've just read the literature that you've provided and I understand it.

GC: There's no nice way to say this but . . . you need to think about the alternatives.

Me: (*seeking clarification*) Do you mean that I should consider having an abortion?

GC: Yes.

Me: I believe that all children are gifts from God, so having an abortion isn't an option for me.

GC: Do you really understand what it means for a child to have CRS?

Me: I do, but being a parent is a privilege and you love the child that you've been blessed with.

GC: What about your husband. What would he think?

Me: We both feel very strongly that all children are precious because they are a gift from God.

(*Here there is a pause for a moment as the 'counsellor' tries to think of a new strategy.*)

GC: Do you realise that it is a lot easier to have an abortion at ten weeks rather than at twelve weeks?

Me: (*horrified by the inference that I would be a kinder mother if I killed my baby today rather than waiting two more weeks, I say in a strong passionate voice*) Are you inferring that I should abort my baby on the off-chance that I might have German measles? What if I haven't contracted German measles? I can't kill my baby on a whim. That would be terrible.

GC: Well if you do keep the baby until you're twelve weeks pregnant, will you see a doctor who specialises in CRS?

Me: (*desperate to escape this nightmare*) Okay, but I'm not having an abortion, because I firmly believe that all people are made in the image of God and therefore, on that basis alone, we are all precious.

(*Another long pause*)

GC: (*with a puzzled look on her face*) Are you making this up? Are you religious?

Me: (*with relief at finally being understood*) Yes – my husband and I are Christians and that is why we believe that God creates people exactly the way that he knows is best. There are some people in this world who are given to us just to teach us how to love. Everyone is valuable because everyone is created equally.

GC: Oh.

After a few more formalities, I flee down the steps of the clinic. I phone my husband and tell him to leave work immediately. I can hardly walk. I'm shaking all over. I start to cry in the middle of the street. I feel sick. What was that? I thought counsellors were supposed to listen and give people choices. She was awful.

Twelve very long days followed. My husband and I talked and talked and talked. We cried. We prayed. It was like we were in our own private world trying to comfort and uphold each other. Our marriage grew stronger and deeper. The threat of CRS and the implications for our family (we had another child who was eighteen months old at the time) were discussed and pondered fully. In all of this, our resolve to protect our unborn child was strengthened. There were no questions in our mind. This baby would be loved.

I'm booked in for the earliest appointment of the day. I have a blood test. I wait until 5 pm and then I phone for the results. I didn't contract German measles! In fact, my rubella reading actually went backwards – it dropped from eight to seven. I really, really didn't get German measles. My baby is perfectly healthy.

I ring my husband immediately to celebrate. The person I ring next is my friend whose child had the German measles. She is most relieved.

On 7 June our beautiful daughter Amelia Grace was born. She is a picture of health and we thank God for her every day.

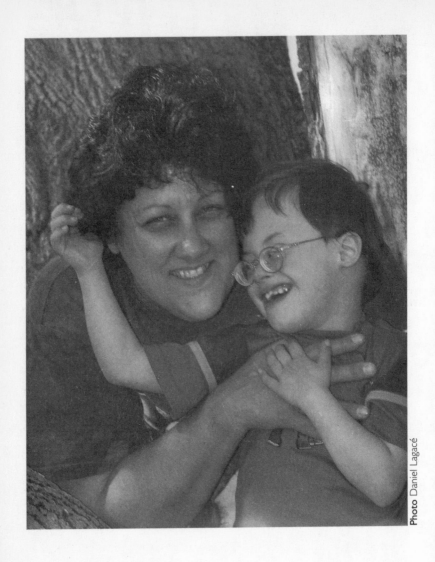

Lise Poirier-Groulx

Dr Lise Poirier-Groulx has been a family physician for almost twenty years. She lives in Ottawa, Canada with her husband François and their children Isabelle (13), Geneviève (9) and Christian (6). In June 2003 she opened the first adult Down syndrome medical clinic in Canada.

Lise Poirier-Groulx

THE BLESSINGS
FAR OUTWEIGH THE SORROWS

Finding myself pregnant at 40 was a total surprise, and somewhat of a shock for my husband of fifteen years. After giving birth to two healthy daughters and suffering a miscarriage, we were not expecting to have any more children. At 34 weeks gestation, I marvelled at the fact that this pregnancy had been my easiest of all with no complications whatsoever. That is, up until then.

At that point I was going for a routine ultrasound to check the baby's position since my first-born had been an undiagnosed breech presentation requiring a caesarean section delivery. Little did I know that that day was going to be the most significant turning point in my life.

I looked forward to seeing my baby on the screen again. The examination lasted longer than usual and I became somewhat concerned, wondering what the problem was. Being a physician myself, I could easily sense the malaise in the room although I could not, with great accuracy, read ultrasound images. The technician discreetly excused herself to get the radiologist to come in and check the image she was seeing. My heart started to race, as well as my mind: 'There has to be something seriously wrong for her to be doing this' I told myself. After what seemed like an eternity but was in fact only ten minutes, a colleague I imme-diately recognised came in to confirm what the technician had suspected. He briefly explained that the ventricles in my baby's brain were enlarged because of too much fluid. I did not believe what I was hearing, and I was convinced that they were wrong. The doctor invited me to his office to discuss the matter further. I followed in a daze, repeating to myself angrily: 'They are wrong; my baby does not have hydrocephalus.'

My colleague, who was obviously quite uncomfortable to be the one giving me this information, was nevertheless very compassionate. He talked in medical jargon, speaking to the doctor in me as the mother's heart in me was breaking. I was having a hard time hearing what he was saying.

I managed to understand that my baby was too small for gestational age, that the amniotic fluid around him was inadequate and that he had hydrocephalus. I called my husband immediately after I came out of the office and, for the first time in my life, I could not talk because I was crying too much. All I could manage to say was that there was something seriously wrong with our baby and that I would explain later.

The following days were a blur as we kept ourselves busy, waiting to have a second more detailed ultrasound to further evaluate our baby.

We were finally given an appointment five days later. I was hoping against hope that all of this was just a mistake, that the results of this second ultrasound would come back normal. Not only were the first results confirmed, but a severe congenital heart malformation incompatible with life outside the womb, was also detected. My head was spinning by then; this was becoming a nightmare that I could not get out of.

The neonatologist brought my husband and I into a private room to talk. She was courteous in explaining that our baby was suffering from a complete outflow tract obstruction, which meant that no blood could be pumped from the heart to the lungs. This was not a problem as long as the fetus remained in the mother's womb where breathing was not necessary to oxygenate the blood.

Most of these cases ended with either the baby dying in utero, or during delivery, or shortly after birth. She continued by saying that she had contacted my gynaecologist and had discussed the results with her; everything could quickly be arranged to terminate the pregnancy. Inducing premature labor on a fetus of one pound with severe multiple congenital birth defects would do what mother nature usually does and had not done in this case. I was shocked. I had not seen this coming. I felt naïve and betrayed.

I did not even need to consider what she was proposing to us because I knew that neither my husband nor I would entertain this possibility. We had made the decision early on in the pregnancy not to undergo the routine amniocentesis because we knew we would not go through with an abortion if the baby had been diagnosed with a handicap. With very few words (as I was stunned) and no justification, I told her so. Her attitude abruptly changed; she became distant and cold. She advised us that she had arranged an urgent prenatal echocardiogram with a pediatric cardiologist at the children's hospital in Ottawa in order to have a precise diagnosis of the heart malformation.

Within half an hour we were seated in the waiting room in the Department of Cardiology. My husband and I spoke very little; the depth of our sadness overwhelmed us.

After the echocardiogram, we met with the cardiologist who explained to us with detailed drawings the two different types of outflow tract obstructions which occur in approximately 1 in 8000 births. They had been unable to identify which one our baby had; the prognosis, however, was the same for both. We again reiterated our choice not to terminate the pregnancy. In view of this, he went on to propose two different scenarios in the event that our baby would be born alive. One was to let nature take its course and not to intervene, in other words enjoy what little time we had with our baby. The second was to give our baby a drug to 'buy time' in order for investigations to be done. Fearing that we would cause unnecessary suffering and knowing that we would still not change the unavoidable outcome of death, we chose the first option.

Next, we were summoned to the geneticist. She told us that an amniocentesis was indicated to attempt to identify a syndrome which could explain the multiple birth defects from which our baby was suffering. We already knew this test could not be performed because there was insufficient amniotic fluid. And for us, in any case, having that extra information would not have changed our decision of going on with the pregnancy. At that time, it was speculated that the most likely diagnosis was either trisomy 13 or trisomy 18. Both these syndromes are comprised of multiple birth defects associated with a very poor prognosis as described previously. Since we insisted we did not want to terminate the pregnancy, the geneticist gave us a pamphlet of testimonies of parents who had gone through what we were about to go through.

It had been an exhausting day to say the least; all we could do now was wait. We decided that we wanted to monitor the baby closely with twice-weekly biophysical profiles in the hope of having a live birth by caesarean section.

Our coping strategy at the time was to concentrate on the present moment; our baby was alive now. We could at least let ourselves enjoy him for whatever time was left. This was extremely difficult as we tried to go on with the task of 'normal' living. Our intense grief was compounded by worries of how we would prepare our two daughters (three-and-a-half and seven at the time) for the death of the baby they had been waiting for all these months. We planned a christening in the operating room and set a date for the funeral one week after the delivery. The four weeks preceding the baby's birth were horrendous for all of us.

The membranes ruptured one week prior to the date set for the caesarean section. With anxious trepidation, we rushed to the hospital. We had paged our doctor, who met us in the delivery room. Everything was arranged with thorough efficiency and we soon found ourselves in the operating room. My husband was given permission to remain by my side for the whole procedure. Without delay, under spinal anesthesia, our baby was delivered. Dead silence prevailed as everyone waited, not daring to move, in order to hear whether this little one would actually take his first breath and cry. To the pediatrician's amazement he was found to be more vigorous than expected, with APGARs (a recording of the physical health of a newborn infant) of 4 and 6, and he weighed 4 lb (1.9 kg) at term, 38 weeks gestation.

As I am writing this, everything is flooding back to me with such intensity: the memories of the first minutes with him, how adorable and fragile he appeared with his tiny cream-colored cap, swaddled warmly so that only his small face was visible. Just looking at him, he seemed so perfect; only his pale purplish skin color hinted at how seriously ill he was. This precious bundle was placed in my husband's arms; I could not move to touch him. Emotions overwhelmed me as I started to cry and felt I would faint. Immediately, I was medicated to help me deal with the whole situation. The christening proceeded as my brother-in-law videotaped every solemn moment; these pictures could be the only memories we had of our baby alive. The atmosphere was thick with apprehension.

My husband followed as our baby was transferred to the neonatal intensive care unit (NICU) in an incubator with 100 percent oxygen. I feared my baby would die before I was able to leave the operating room and before I could see him again and hopefully hold him.

After barely an hour in the recovery room, I was brought to the neonatal unit. As I saw my son Christian, so vulnerable, lying in his incubator with the different monitoring equipment attached to him, I was overcome with love. I could not have enough of stroking him. It was so hard, lying on my stretcher, reaching to touch him through the openings of the incubator. Seeing my predicament, a compassionate nurse broke protocol and took him out of his sterile environment and placed him gently into my arms. I was so grateful for her gesture, tears flooded my face as I kissed my little one. The time was too short. He had to be transferred to a tertiary care centre. I had to let him go. The fear of losing him, the fear of the decisions to be made, the fear of the unknown, was overwhelming.

Because Christian appeared so much stronger than expected, we reconsidered our initial plan and decided to go ahead with the second scenario, which was to treat him with a drug called prostaglandin. It tricks the heart into thinking that it is still in the mother's womb. In doing so it 'buys time' to investigate further and if possible do cardiac surgery. Because of the risk of serious side-effects, it could only be used for one week.

The echocardiogram revealed the heart anomaly to be Tetralogy of Fallot with pulmonary atresia. In lay terms, it means there were four major problems with his heart:

1. the malformation of the pulmonary trunk leading to both pulmonary arteries prevented any blood from going from the heart to the lungs;
2. a large hole existed between the two lower chambers of the heart;
3. the aorta (which carries blood from the heart to the rest of the body) was in the wrong position;
4. the right lower chamber wall was too thick and therefore not contracting well enough to pump blood.

An ultrasound of his head revealed no evidence of hydrocephalus (in my denial, I had been right after all!). A chromosomal study revealed trisomy 21 (Down syndrome). Although this information was hard to take, it was still better news than what we had been given during the pregnancy. We decided to go ahead with surgery.

Christian was nine days old when a right classic B-T shunt was performed. An artery from his right arm was reversed in order for blood to be 'shunted' from the heart to the lungs to bypass the malformation of the pulmonary trunk or outflow tract. Although he came through the surgery, the procedure was not a success.

Twenty-one days later a central aorto-pulmonary shunt was performed successfully and the outcome was above and beyond the cardiologist's expectations.

Christian spent eight-and-a-half months of his first year in hospital. He underwent four major surgeries during that time: three for his heart and one for his stomach (reflux problem). He was in and out of intensive care and spent the greater part of his time on the surgical ward in an oxyhood (similar to an oxygen tent). At ten-and-a-half months of age, he was finally transferred to Toronto Sick Children's Hospital, where he had a total repair of his heart. This included the use of a human tissue graft from a donor to replace the malformed pulmonary trunk or outflow tract. His recovery was truly miraculous, as witnessed by the doctors and nurses.

He has needed seven cardiac catheterizations for diverse medical reasons since then. Although he requires continuous medical follow-up, he has surpassed all expectations in regards to his growth, development and his quality of life.

Christian is now six years of age. He started school in August 2004. What a celebration that was – we never thought he would make it that far! He is presently totally asymptomatic from a cardiac standpoint and does not take any cardiac medications. It is expected that he will require further cardiac surgery in order to replace the human tissue graft, which will not grow as he grows up. He is a very loving, happy, active little boy who continually gets himself into trouble and annoys his older sisters. They both adore him.

Although the journey has been incredibly difficult for the entire family, we have absolutely no regrets. The blessings which accompanied this little one into our lives far outweigh the sorrows we have experienced. We have grown and learned so very much through him. Every day, we witness how he touches people's hearts, and people's lives are changed just because of who he is. Everyone who knows him loves him!

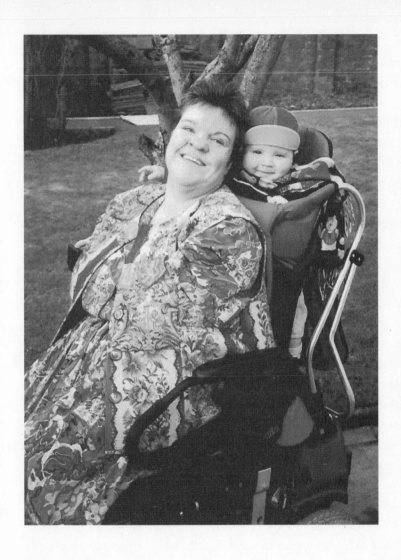

Rosaleen Moriarty-Simmonds

Rosaleen Moriarty-Simmonds lives in Cardiff, South Wales (UK), with her husband Stephen and son James. Writing this piece has revived her passion for the written word and she now intends to fulfil one of her ambitions by writing her autobiography: Four fingers and thirteen toes.

Rosaleen Moriarty-Simmonds

JUST CRASH THROUGH IT

I am a 44-year-old disabled woman, a happy wife, an adoring mum, a successful businesswoman, a school governor, a voluntary worker, an artist, and a socialite – constantly busy and totally content. I was born and bred in Cardiff, South Wales. My parents are of Irish origin; Dad comes from Ardfert, outside Tralee and my late mother came from Ballyhack, a small fishing village in Wexford, near Waterford. I have two younger sisters, Deborah and Denise. Most people call me Rosie.

My impairment is 'four limbed phocomelia', caused by the drug Thalidomide. Basically, I have little legs which end above the knee (similar to an amputee) but with feet, and from each shoulder I have two fingers. Further, I have sight loss in my left eye, and hearing loss in my right ear. I do not know what internal organs were damaged, if any, because I have never been checked/body scanned, and I do not have a particular desire to find out anyway.

Thalidomide is a non-barbiturate hypnotic drug first discovered in Germany in 1954. By 1957 it was actively marketed there and in many other countries throughout the world to treat surprisingly minor ailments such as colds, coughs and flu. By the time it was withdrawn in Germany on 27 November 1961, Thalidomide was marketed under 51 names, in 11 European, seven African, 17 Asian and 11 American countries.

The drug was first marketed in Britain in April 1958, by Distillers Company (Biochemicals) Limited (subject to a takeover by Guinness in 1986 and subsequently by Deagio) under the names Thalidomide, Distaval, Tensival, Asmaval, Valgis and Valgraine. For two years it was available over the counter as well as by prescription. Thalidomide was promoted widely as the 'wonder drug', and just prior to its withdrawal in the UK, Distillers were actively marketing Thalidomide, even with literature stressing how safe the drug was: 'without any risk to mother or child'.

If Thalidomide was taken throughout the sensitive period of pregnancy, i.e. the first three months, and then between day 35 and day 49, the consequences were generally severe defects of ears, arms and legs and internal malformations, which often led to early death. There were 12,000 Thalidomide-impaired babies born world-wide. About another 40 percent of them died before their first birthday.

Like many women, my mother suffered with severe morning sickness, and as a result, the family doctor prescribed Thalidomide to alleviate the symptoms. Pregnancy scanning did not exist in the late 1950s and early 1960s, so nobody knew that my mother was carrying a disabled child until I was born on 6 December 1960.

My mother had already been in hospital for about a month with toxaemia, and consequently she had come to know the doctors and nurses quite well. She had to be induced, and when I was finally born I was taken away abruptly and my mother was just left there on her own on the birthing table. She was barely 18 years of age! I remember her telling me that she had assumed I was stillborn because of the reactions of the midwife and doctors. With hindsight, she recalled that they had looked shocked and distressed, muttered frantically, and then the nurse disappeared with me in her arms. Eventually, somebody came and just sedated my mum.

Apparently none of the doctors and nurses from the maternity hospital felt able to tell my father what had happened when he arrived at the hospital after work. Another doctor was called over from the main hospital, and he had the difficult task of trying to explain to my dad what the situation was. But frustratingly he did not have the answers to my father's many questions. When my dad later returned to my grandparents' house where a number of relatives were waiting to find out if mum had had a girl or a boy, he apparently had to be held down because he just lost it. He was so grief-stricken and unable to comprehend what had happened, how, or why.

For many years he and my mother carried a terrible burden of self-blame and pity. We talked about the situation occasionally, and no matter how many times I told them, 'I do not blame you', you could still see the sadness behind their eyes.

Three days after I was born my mother pulled out the sedation drip and tried to make her way to the nursery. Before she could get there she collapsed and haemorrhaged. Eventually, the doctors realised that they had to try and explain to my mum what had happened, and let her see me. So they wrapped me up and handed me to her. Initially, as with all babies wrapped up, all you can see is their little face looking up at you. In her own time mum unwrapped the blanket. It did not seem to matter to her that I did not have any arms or legs. We fell in love with each other instantly and an unbreakable bond between mother and daughter was formed. She told me that she said, 'Isn't she beautiful; she's all mine.' From that moment on I was treated like every other member of the family. Whatever physical, attitudinal or environmental barriers we came across, it was as a family. Wherever the family went, I went also. This was despite the doctors saying to my parents, 'You are a young couple; leave her here [at the hospital], go away and start all over again.' Thankfully, my parents were horrified and, as young as they were, they were adamant I was going home with them. They were both brought up as strict

Catholics, and had the support of an extended family. We all moved in with my maternal grandparents, and I was much loved by everyone.

I was one of the lucky ones; roughly 50 percent of the Thalidomide-impaired babies born in this country were abandoned by their parents to be brought up in 'hospital homes'. Thalidomide affected the parents, the families and the Thalidomide-impaired child on a totally arbitrary basis – rich and poor; road sweepers and scientists; across cultures and religions. Some parents divorced because an agreement could not be reached on the child's destiny. For those families who decided to keep their Thalidomide-impaired child, most siblings were protective and loving, though others saw their Thalidomide-impaired brother or sister as an intrusion or rival, particularly if the disabled child needed a lot of physical help.

I was always encouraged to be as independent as possible, to stand up for my rights and the rights of others, to speak up and be heard, to 'never say never', to believe that there is no such word as 'can't'. In fact, a good friend of mine, also Thalidomide-impaired (who has since passed away), and myself came up with this wonderful motto: 'If you can't get over it, or you can't get around it, you just crash through it.'

There were over 450 Thalidomide-impaired babies born who survived in this country between 1958 and 1962. And the medical profession got excited. They had a whole host of guinea pigs on which to experiment. Their attitude at the time was, if bits are missing, replace them. Generally, society's perception of 'image, beauty and normality' has been influenced throughout history, going back to the Greek and Roman ideas of 'the body beautiful'. To make us more acceptable-looking, more 'normal'-looking to the rest of society so that society would accept us, the medics would have to replace the missing bits. So I, like many others, had numerous operations to straighten my legs (which were coiled round and lying flat on my stomach at birth). It would have been commendable had they left it at that, but instead, what followed was being fitted with artificial limbs or prosthetics. I spent hours of painful and frustrating rehabilitation trying to learn to walk on the artificial legs; a bit of a futile exercise really, particularly if you don't have arms with which to balance or protect yourself when you fall. Then came the artificial arms, attached to a little metal jacket, powered by a gas cylinder on your back; yet again more rehabilitation. Because we were falling over on a regular basis, it was decided to give us crash helmets as well. Far from looking 'normal', which was of course, the intention, we ended up looking like Metal Mickey!

What they hadn't noticed (despite film footage in my medical records) was that, left to my own devices and the little bits I had, I could do a lot better, a lot quicker, in my own way and with a smile on my face!

My family gave me every opportunity to develop to my fullest potential. However trying to get a good and meaningful education was more of a struggle. Between the ages of 4 and 14 I went to a school for disabled children, which was a taxi ride from home. In the 1960s not much was expected from disabled people and consequently you were not expected to leave school with any qualifications. The school I was at had a mixed bunch of children with varying abilities, from those with learning difficulties, to others with mental health issues, and children with physical impairments like myself. The whole school went at the pace of the slowest; we had a good social life, and were taken many places on the 'big green bus', but we did not achieve academically.

It was not until 1970 that the education legislation in the UK was changed to include disabled children. At long last disabled people had a right to be educated. Around about this time a new headmaster came to the school. He had a meeting with my parents which was pivotal in shaping my academic future. Up until then, my parents had met with a brick wall as far as the education authorities were concerned. Even the local infants and junior school, which my sister Deborah (younger by sixteen months) attended, did not know of my existence. We learnt this one day when my mum went to pick Deborah up from school, only to find her in floods of tears. The children in her class had been asked to tell a story about somebody that they admired. She talked about her elder sister, who didn't have any arms or legs, and Deborah was told off by the teacher for having 'a horrible imagination!' This quite vividly portrays the attitude of society towards disabled people in the 1960s.

In February 1975, I found myself at an all-girls boarding school – Florence Treloar School, in Alton, Hampshire. At that time it was the only school in the country for disabled people which offered an education at grammar school level. The previously mentioned headmaster saw my potential and pulled a few strings to assist me to gain a place at the school. I am privileged to have gone there; we were given so many opportunities. I excelled and in three years caught up and achieved a number of qualifications.

I then went on to Hereward College in Coventry, again for disabled people. I attained a Business Education Council General qualification, and some more O levels. We had a lot of independence at college, a great social life, and freedom to date the boys!

In September 1980 I finally got to attend a mainstream college at home here in Cardiff, where I again did business studies (the careers advisers had no imagination!). For the first time ever, I finally realised that academically I was an equal with my non-disabled fellow students.

Fed up with business studies, and having spent most of my life observing the behaviour of other people, I went to Cardiff

University and graduated in 1985 with a degree in Psychology.

After graduating, I naïvely thought it would be a doddle getting a job. What a shock! Despite sending over 250 job applications, I ended up with only four interviews. Eventually, this culminated in me getting a job in the civil service as an Executive Officer (at middle management level). I had intended to only stay for a couple of years to get some experience under my belt. Seven years later, I accepted a voluntary redundancy package. I spent most of 1993 doing a journalism course and at the same time got more involved in the disabled people's movement and trained to become a disability equality trainer. However, by 1995 work had taken off at such a pace that I established the RMS Disability Issues Consultancy, which offers large and small organisations in the private and public sector either consultancy on disability issues or training (primarily disability equality training and training around legislation like the Disability Discrimination Act 1995).

I first laid eyes on the man who would become my husband when we were 4 or 5 years old, at the limb-fitting centre in the Prudential Buildings, Cardiff (now the Hilton Hotel). We continued to bump into each other there until we were in our teens and also at the Thalidomide Society AGM and conference meetings. In our early twenties a number of Thalidomide-impaired people living in Wales decided that it was a shame that we only met up once a year at the Thalidomide Society weekends, so we started to meet in a pub or restaurant, roughly once a month. This fizzled out, but Stephen and I kept in touch fairly regularly as friends.

By our mid-twenties we had both graduated and settled into permanent jobs – Stephen as a solicitor and me as a civil servant. Out of the blue, Stephen phoned me at work one day to invite me to the opening of a restaurant for which he had done some work. We had both been in relationships with other people, but were single at that time. We had a lovely night out and I found myself thinking, 'He's a good looking fellow, and he has a lovely personality, so why not . . . ?' It was the start of a whirlwind romance in which I discovered that Stephen had loved me for many years, but had not said so, for fear of spoiling the very good friendship that we had enjoyed. We got engaged in May 1987 and married in September 1988.

Looking back, I remember at around the age of 12 or 13, while on one of many stays at the rehabilitation unit of the Nuffield Orthopaedic Hospital in Oxford, one of the nurses took me and another good friend who was Thalidomide-impaired (who has also since passed away), to one side and tried to explain to us about the facts of life. We spent most of the time giggling out of embarrassment and almost missed the point that she was trying to make, which was basically that because our bodies were unique, and because the medical profession did not know how our bodies were going to develop, they could not say for certain whether or not we would be able to have children.

Like most girls, I wanted to grow up, get married, have a family and live happily ever after. But once I had been told that I may not be able to have children, and not being one who particularly likes to experience pain, I went through a period of believing that babies were not for me. But soon after Stephen and I married, my sister Deborah had her daughter Jodie, my friend Tina had Kerry, and my maternal clock kicked in.

Now and then members of the medical profession, total strangers, and once or twice even family members expressed the view that I probably wouldn't be able to have children, and some even said I shouldn't. They were making lots of assumptions about me medically, and were perhaps concerned that having a baby might affect my health. For anyone else who even fleetingly thought ill of my ability to look after a child or organise the looking after of my child, then, two fingers to them – literally!

Typically, when you really want something it doesn't come easy. We tried for two years and nothing happened. We tried temperature charts, nothing happened. Eventually, after a grilling from the doctors at the infertility centre – 'Are you sure? How will you manage? Your health may be affected, etc etc' – I tried a mild fertility drug.

I had three miscarriages, two at 8 weeks, and the third at 10 weeks. Each time we were heartbroken. With all the progress in medical science, they were unable to tell us the reasons for the miscarriages.

We got to the stage of having to think about IVF and so took time out to give it some consideration. Whilst trying to think what to do next and trying to come to terms with the prospect of being a childless couple, the miracle happened.

Just before Christmas 1994 we discovered that I was pregnant again. We were both ecstatic and petrified. Ecstatic, because it had happened without any help! Petrified, because I had lost my three other babies and was worried that the same could happen again. As a result, apart from our GP who was fantastic both in attitude and support, we told nobody else until after I had passed 12 weeks.

Some family members were concerned when we told them, others were delighted, friends were pleased and strangers – when they came to know – were shocked, surprised, curious or pleased. We encountered lots of questions, anything from, 'How did you get pregnant?' We would reply, 'Well, if you don't know now, you will never know!' 'I guess you will have to stay in bed for the whole nine months?' Answer: 'I hope not, I have a business to run'. 'What about your health?' Answer; 'I am not ill, I am having a baby, I look and feel healthier now than ever.' 'How will you manage?' 'Who will look after the baby?' and so on.

We had all the answers; we had had a long time to think about it. We watched how other people looked after their children and worked out exactly how we would manage at every stage, what gadgets, or equipment, or physical support from others we might need to invent, obtain or purchase. Most people look at salad tongs, for example, and see only one use for them; disabled people looked at salad tongs and see several uses for them.

Because Stephen and I were both born Thalidomide-impaired, we have spent all our lives finding ways to manage in everyday situations. We had already achieved so much: we were well educated, loved by our families, learnt to drive adapted cars, got married, got good jobs, and then went on to run our own businesses, run our own home and have a great social life; bringing up a child was going to be a doddle after all that!

If anybody frowned on our decision to have a child, as usual they have been proven wrong.

I must have been born to be 'Mother Earth', and I think under other circumstances I would have had lots of children. Throughout my pregnancy I blossomed. Obviously I got more tired as the pregnancy went on; naturally I got wider! As a consequence I had to do physical things like getting on and off the toilet and in and out of bed more slowly. But I worked right up until two weeks before James was born.

The medical support I had during my pregnancy was shared between my GP and the Maternity Department at our local hospital. Interestingly, my GP said he would make sure that I was to be passed to a professor at the hospital who was 'more open-minded'. I understood the point that he was making: even in this day and age there are still people, particularly in the medical profession, who actually believe that disabled people should not have children.

On our first visit to the hospital, I made it clear that I was not going to have any intrusive examinations, neither was I going to allow them to take blood to do the tests to see if I was carrying a disabled child or not. Both Stephen and I (who are poles apart as far as disability politics is concerned) agreed that even if we did have a disabled child, it did not matter, we would still love and cherish it. Further, because I had already had three miscarriages, I did not want to risk losing this baby. The biggest surprise of that visit came when I met the senior midwife. It turned out that she had been a junior nurse on duty on the day that I was born at the Glossop Maternity Hospital. We talked about the impact that my birth had had on so many people. She was sorry to hear that my mother had passed away, but she was delighted that I was pregnant and endeavoured to make sure that my pregnancy and birthing experience was going to be a positive one.

Exactly on the day expected, just after I had waddled on to the toilet at 8 am on 9 August 1995, my waters broke. I remember thinking, 'Lucky it happened while on the toilet, if it had happened whilst still in my electric wheelchair, it might have short circuited!'

Stephen came home from work and we arrived at the hospital mid-morning. Although my waters had broken there was not a single sign of a contraction. The professor I was under was an advocate of natural births and although I quite fancied the idea of being knocked out and then later handed a nice clean pink baby, he had other ideas. By mid-afternoon they induced me and the contractions came hard and fast. By 6 pm the following night and several different shifts of midwives, I had only dilated four centimetres, I was exhausted, distressed and worried about my baby. Eventually, they decided to do an emergency caesarean.

There were only two other Thalidomide-impaired women with almost identical impairments to mine that I knew of who had had children – both of them had had caesareans so I was not shocked, but more angry with myself for not having insisted on an 'elective caesarean' in the first place.

Right up until this moment I had been treated with respect and no distinction made between me and all the other mums at the antenatal classes and clinics. I was given my own room because it was recognised that I would need more privacy and support, and an air of excitement and anticipation buzzed around the hospital. But then the duty anaesthetist arrived. I have seldom encountered anyone more ignorant and rude. He stood leaning against the radiator, with his back to the window, muttering into the ground and refusing to make eye contact. I explained that I could not hear what he was saying. I asked him to stand at the foot of my bed so that I could hear better; he just ignored me. At that point Stephen blew his top. The anaesthetist was supposed to be explaining his intentions of giving me an epidural, but with all the baby monitors and other noisy equipment and because he was muttering, I did not have a clue what was going on.

Eventually, after his numerous failed attempts at trying to give me an epidural, a more senior anaesthetist was called in and after lying on the theatre bed for over an hour, being prodded and poked like a pincushion, he managed to get a drip into my neck. James was born by caesarean at 8:42 pm on Thursday 10 August 1995, weighing 7 lb 2 oz. Later that night I was handed a nice clean pink baby!

Although I was pretty much out of it when they first put James by my face, I recall this beautiful little face with big blue eyes looking at me and I said 'Hello James, my beautiful little boy', and then I blanked out again.

The next day when we were back on the regular ward and he was in the little see-through plastic cot looking out at me, all I could do was look straight back at him. He was absolutely gorgeous and fascinating and the love I felt for him was instant and intense. That warm glow of pride, love and devotion only a mother can feel, mixed with the ferocious desire to protect, nurture and treasure. Nature and instinct are incredible things – this normally wriggly little bundle of fun instantly relaxed when he was placed on me for a cuddle, or when I held or carried him.

Seven days after James was born we arrived home to a house full of flowers, cards and good wishes from family, friends and acquaintances.

We soon settled into the routine of feeding, winding, bathing, changing, playing, cuddling, sleeping. The only thing I could not do for James but could supervise, was bathe him. The one thing I chose to delegate, was changing dirty nappies – having only two fingers from the shoulders means my face was just a little too close to the nappy for comfort! We were well organised; we had thought and planned everything through in advance. For example, we brought a cot that had one side that went right down to the floor for easy access to James; had a nappy changing unit made to our requirements; car seat times two, one for my car, one for Steve's; a dozen bottles, long thin ones or the 'Nipper gripper' type, which I found easier to handle – we would make up six bottles at a time and the others would then be sterilising ready to be made up the next evening. Two of the most useful pieces of equipment were a portable baby seat, which we strapped on to the dining-room chair so that James could sit at the table with us wherever we were and in which I could initially feed him until he was able to feed himself. The second useful piece of equipment was a backpack baby carrier, the kind that athletic parents use to carry their babies on their back. I strapped this to the back of my electric wheelchair, James was then strapped into the backpack and everybody was happy – particularly James because he could see where we were going and when he was tired, he could fall asleep on my shoulder.

When I bottle fed him I laid him flat out on the dining-room table. When he was on solids and in the high chair, I cellotaped two long plastic spoons together to make one long one, I would put the handle end in my mouth, scoop up the food, and put it in James's mouth.

We employed a 'Mothers Help' (alias 'Aunty Anne') a couple of days a week to help me look after James when Stephen was at work. I had used voice control to stop James harming himself while crawling and walking, but could not guarantee that this would work when we were out walking. So I bought some reins for him, only to discover that the strap was not long enough. Then I had the bright idea of attaching a retractable dog lead to the rein's strap. This allowed James enough freedom and I had the security of knowing that I still had control.

The only downside to this was that there were actually members of the public who said things like 'Oh how cute, is he pulling you along then?' And, 'He's a strong little chappy to be able to pull you along like that!' My stock answer through gritted teeth and a false smile, would be: 'Yes, it's a new Winter Olympics sport, babies pulling sledges through the snow and I'm training him up!' It was usually worth it just to see their expressions. However, there was one comment that really used to rile me, and that was 'I bet he is your arms and legs'. No, absolutely not. He was not put on this earth to be my slave and other people even thinking or implying that makes me so angry. I am vehemently against children being expected to look after their disabled parents. Don't get me wrong, making their bed, tidying away their toys, helping to lay the table should be expected of children in every household. But expecting children to lift, dress, toilet, bath, feed and give 24 hour support to a disabled parent is, in my opinion, wholly wrong and unfair on the child.

Generally, when James was a baby, then as a toddler, and now as a typical 9-year-old out and about with his disabled parents, the reaction of members of the public is warm and positive. It can range from total indifference to quizzical curiosity and James handles this in a polite and mature way. Occasionally, if people stare, James has been known to pull a face at them, and if people ask him probing questions, he has been known to come back with an equally outrageous answer. For example, once when asked why his mum didn't have any arms or legs, he answered 'She fell into the lion's cage!'

James and I have a wonderful mother and son relationship – open, honest, affectionate and loving. We cuddle, kiss and tell each other 'I love you' numerous times throughout the day. James is sporty, musical, artistic, very bright and extremely popular. Whatever James wants to do, we have always encouraged and helped him – like all parents it's usually acting as a taxi driver. James will grow up to be a well balanced, thoughtful, hard-working adult with a fantastic personality. I am proud to say that I have had some small part in that.

In the early days when we were children and teenagers, the medical profession had very few expectations of the abilities and capabilities of Thalidomide-impaired people. Including being uncertain as to whether or not, we would be able to have children. When in later years many of us went on to do so, any negative responses tended to be more social and or practical ones, rather than medical. The fact that there are now more children of Thalidomide-impaired parents, than there are Thalidomide-impaired people, speaks for itself in many ways.

It further reinforces the fact that Thalidomide-impaired people have been the protagonists of the disabled people's movement. We have bulldozed our way through many of the barriers that society puts in the way of disabled people – the majority of us just quietly get on with their lives without our impairment being the main issue. We have used our strengths to bring about many changes in legislation and social policy. Generally society has become more accepting of seeing disabled people as a direct result of the Thalidomide story. Until this event, the majority of disabled people were accommodated in institutions, hospitals and other establishments away from the public eye. Horrific injuries, often caused by the ravages of the Two World Wars, were perceived as being too distressing for public view. This changed when many of the parents of Thalidomide children refused to allow their children to be seen as objects of pity, and were proud to be seen with their children as a whole family unit.

Life as a Thalidomide impaired woman at this moment in time is good, as far as I am concerned. I am a confident woman, I am in control of my life, I have a wonderful husband, a fabulous son, a successful business, a comfortable home, a good social life, loyal friends, I am respected and my opinions are sought. But it has not always been that way, and there are still very many Thalidomide-impaired and other disabled women who still encounter negative attitudes and discrimination.

I have in my lifetime experienced discrimination, and negative attitudes – usually from ignorant, ill-informed people who were probably totally oblivious to their behaviour. I have been thrown out of two shops, denied access to cinemas and nightclubs, talked about as if I were invisible, denied jobs because of being disabled, been physically abused, had incorrect assumptions made about me, been stared at – and the list goes on.

I coped with the bad things and experiences, because mostly I had good things and good experiences and good people around me. Generally, I have a bubbly, confident personality, which sees me through the bad things. With a sense of humour, you can usually turn a negative thing around to see the funny side of it, and if you can laugh at yourself and the situation in which you find yourself – then you have cracked it.

When people stare at me – I smile at them. If people are rude, ignorant or mean to me, I either challenge them or ignore them. If people are obviously discriminating towards me, and they are in breach of legislation or not even prepared to implement best practice, then I definitely confront them, point out the error and do my best to change their attitude or the situation.

In an ideal world, non-disabled women and disabled women alike would be able to bring a child into a society that does not discriminate against disabled people – sadly, we do not live in an ideal world. We live in a world where there is prejudice against and fear of disabled people, where there are powerful and negative influences against a woman being able to make an informed decision regarding the future of the child that she is carrying. It concerns me that prenatal testing, and therapeutic abortion are offered in an almost mandatory way, the prejudicial availability of these procedures only seeks to limit women's choice.

Regrettably, there are still people – mostly in the medical profession – who are strongly against disabled women having children. To them, and society in general, I say society has to change to include disabled people. The structures and barriers within society have to change, i.e. the attitudinal barriers (images of, perceptions of and behaviour towards disabled people), environmental barriers (inaccessible buildings, inaccessible transport, inaccessible information), structural barriers (timetables, rules and regulations, traditional ways, etc.) and other barriers (not being able to access a meaningful education, preferably in mainstream schools, means that disabled people will not be able to access worthwhile and well-paid jobs).

Disabled people have skills that the majority of non-disabled people lack. Disabled women, in particular, are incredibly organised, motivated, proficient, talented, competent and experts in many areas. Disabled women make wonderful mothers, because we have a deep understanding of other people's feelings (particularly children), we have good sense of fun and humour, we are protective of those we love, and we are capable of finding all sorts of innovative ways around any obstacles or barriers that we may come across.

As far as I'm concerned, the positives and rewards of having children far outweigh the negatives.

My only sadness since having James is that my mother was not alive to see him. She died suddenly and tragically on 12 February 1992, at the young age of 49. When she died, part of me died too. I had confided in her that I desperately wanted a baby. She told me I would make a wonderful mother and, philosophical as always, said that if I was meant to have child it would happen. I am fully convinced that she got together with all of the other angels in heaven and answered my prayers to her, by sending James to me. We had a wonderful relationship, very open, very honest, very affectionate, utter devotion and lots of laughs. I only hope that I will be as good a mother to James as my mother was to me.

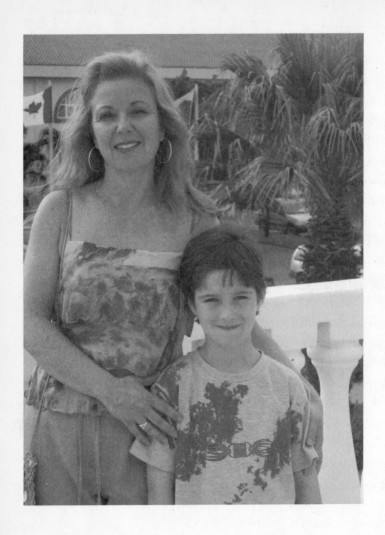

Lisa Roche

Lisa E. Roche is an attorney specialising in probate and consumer law. She lives in York, Maine, USA, with her husband and son. Lisa describes herself as a big fan of Celtic, Blues, R& B, Rock and Jazz. She introduced her son to the Beatles Anthology while in her womb, and it remains his favourite music.

Lisa Roche

GO WITH YOUR INSTINCTS

When I was a teenage girl my biggest problem was that I was a terrible asthmatic. There was no such thing as an inhaler or a 24 hour allergy pill. My remedy was a dose of Tedral. This medication was basically like speed mixed with some bronchial dilator medicine. The tablet tasted like poison and caused my heart to beat so fast and hard that more often than not the remedy did not seem any better than gasping with all my might for each breath, day in, day out. An asthma attack could last a week and then it would take a week to recuperate from the sore arms, ribs and back caused by the attack.

After years of fighting these severe asthma attacks, my body was in no condition to reproduce. I was told some time between 14 and 16 years of age that I suffered from 'non-ovulation' and that is why I still hadn't had my first period. I was told I was infertile and would most likely never have children. I knew the diagnosis was correct because I never did get my period.

At first I was in a state of shock when I realised I would never be a mom – that I would never have a baby. I was only a teenage girl but I understood how this would make my life very different from most other young women. I decided to instead think about a good career. After high school I went to Suffolk University in Boston (USA), and then to Suffolk University Law School. After graduation I started my own solo general legal practice.

From my teens through my twenties I was seriously ill from the combination of asthma attacks and the physical effects of non-ovulation. I would discharge a black substance – dried blood – for anywhere from two weeks to three months. Then I could go for nine months without any discharge. I was only 5 feet 1 inch and weighed about 100 pounds. The constant illnesses wore me down. My doctors always warned me that if I didn't take the birth control pill I would eventually get cervical or ovarian cancer. They said the pill would force my body to have a cycle.

I resisted taking the pill when I was first diagnosed with non-ovulation. My mother, a nurse, was well informed of its dangers and refused to allow it to be my treatment in my teens. When I was in my twenties I took the pill on and off for about ten years because of my fear of cervical and ovarian cancer as well as my fatigue in dealing with the never-ending 'spotting'. But after taking it for a couple of years I thought I would rather have spotting than an emotional roller coaster ride every month due to huge amounts of hormones being pushed into my system. Many doctors refused to have me as a patient because I continued to take myself off the pill during those years, only to return later seeking another prescription.

When my husband Michael and I were first getting serious, dating and talking about plans of marriage, I told him about my diagnosis of infertility. This was a risk. The last man I shared that information with when we were as close could not accept it, and the relationship ended. Although I risked that with Michael, I had to tell him. He had the right to know.

When we talked about getting married and not being able to have children, Michael was not concerned. He accepted it and we moved on and got married.

We decided to celebrate our fifth wedding anniversary with a trip to a warm Caribbean island and go scuba diving, just like we had done on our honeymoon. We chose Jamaica – we had heard the diving was beautiful.

We flew to Jamaica and immediately signed up with the dive shop at the hotel for the next day's dive trip.

On that first morning we went through our pre-dive plan and equipment. After we prepared for two dives that day, we headed for the dive boat. It is normal to feel 'butterflies' in your stomach before a dive. Your life is at risk. As we walked with our dive bags to the boat I began to feel a sense of nervousness that was typical before a first dive. But as I got closer and closer to the boat I began to feel very, very nervous, more so than ever before. I tried to figure out if I was feeling the same pre-dive excitement I usually felt or if I was more nervous than usual. By the time we got to the boat I was slightly panic-stricken. I told Michael I was feeling really scared and didn't know if I wanted to go. Without hesitation he said 'No problem, let's take our names off today's dive trip and sign up for tomorrow. We have all week!' I felt so relieved. We signed up for the next day's trip and went to the pool.

The next morning we got up and went through our pre-dive plan, checked the equipment and headed for the dive boat. It was a gorgeous day. As we approached the boat I once again felt that sudden, uneasy, scared feeling, but it was twice as strong as the day before. This was an unavoidable feeling and the message was clear: 'Don't go.' I knew you should never dive if there is any doubt or uneasiness. Scuba diving is a very dangerous sport and must only be done with total confidence. Michael taught me this lesson and was standing by me when I whispered again under my breath, 'I don't feel right; I don't know if I want to go.' Again, Michael said, without any hesitation, 'No problem. We can still sign up for tomorrow.'

Every day that week we ended up preparing for our dive and walking over to the boat but then rescheduling for the following day. Michael and I never did go diving in Jamaica.

After I was home a few weeks, I had an annual appointment with my obstetrician/gynaecologist. She examined me and discovered

I was about three months pregnant. I was thrilled, overwhelmed, scared and experienced so many other emotions! If I had gone diving, probably down to 100 feet or below, the pressure change would have forced our unborn baby out or would have killed our baby from nitrogen poisoning, commonly known as 'the bends'. Our baby could have been miscarried under the water due to the pressure at that depth. I probably would have panicked, not knowing what was going on, and may have drowned. Thinking that I could have gone diving and killed our baby and me was almost too much to bear. I was so glad that I listened to the little voice inside that simply said 'Don't go!'

But it seemed our baby was still not safe. My obstetrician/gynaecologist had been treating me for several years for non-ovulation and had often rebuked me when I would ask her to let me go off the pill for a while just to see what happened. She seemed to think that I should have accepted my infertility and enjoyed my career and sexual freedom. She could not seem to understand why I would keep considering the possibility of future childbirth.

The fact that I was pregnant seemed to annoy her. Since I had just recently succeeded in persuading her to allow me to stop the pill for six months and do some tests, and then became pregnant, she seemed far from jubilant about my pregnancy.

Although she didn't know my true number of weeks of gestation – because I didn't have a date for a last menstrual period – she estimated I was three months pregnant and took blood for the triple screening test. This test was to screen for Down syndrome, among other conditions.

Within 24 hours of the blood being drawn, my doctor called to let me know that the blood test results had come back and, based on the very low numbers, our baby was going to suffer from severe Down syndrome. She delivered the news in a tone that seemed to say, 'I told you being fertile and having children was not as wonderful as you thought.'

She suggested Michael and I discuss what we 'wanted to do'. I told her that we would not need to discuss that because we would be having our baby regardless of any health conditions. She insisted that we seek counselling before the birth in order to 'cope' with our new lifestyle when our baby was born. She also suggested I have an amniocentesis in order to gain more information and help us to decide what to do. I said again that we would not need an amniocentesis either. She disagreed with my decisions and made me feel I was making poor choices. However, I didn't want to change doctors now, and thought it would be best to keep her rather than find a new doctor in the state to which we had just moved. Later I realised that was a mistake. I should have found a doctor who supported our decisions and helped us celebrate our baby's birth.

Michael researched the triple screening test and learned that the results were only accurate if the blood test is given knowing the actual weeks of gestation. The test had to be administered at an exact time in the pregnancy. There was no way my doctor knew the actual gestation of our baby and whether the test results were reliable, yet she informed me in a very matter-of-fact way that we had a problem. While she could have been right, I didn't like the way she came across as so certain that she was right.

I was excited about having a baby but I was also very worried about what our future lifestyle would be like with our child. I was also concerned that perhaps we would have a baby with severe Down syndrome. It would be difficult, but I believed we would make the best of it for our family.

The days leading up to the delivery date of 28 December were long and worrisome. I kept trying to figure out which way it would be for us. Then 28 December came and went and not one contraction. Then 29, and 30, and 31 December, and New Years! By 3 January it was decided that I should be induced. I spent the entire day and night in the hospital but no results. We had to go home and then return on 5 January for a second attempt at inducing labor.

I was finally induced and had my waters broken a few hours later. I had begun hard labor when I was told my doctor would not be in for the delivery but that her partner would handle it. Our son Brady Jude Roche was born at 1:15 am, 6 January in one of the worst blizzards ever to hit New England.

I anxiously waited for the pediatrician to give him his first medical examination. The pediatrician was extremely annoyed because he had had to come out in the snowstorm. This man behaved in the most unprofessional, uncaring, rude manner. When I asked what Brady's APGAR score was, he yelled, 'You can't rely on that; it doesn't tell you anything!' He then begrudgingly stated that Brady had scored a nine on the APGAR test. A nurse in the maternity ward overheard the way the doctor spoke to me and reported him to the head of the hospital. Later that day the hospital administrator apologised for the pediatrician's unprofessional conduct and misinformation on the reliability of the APGAR score. She informed me my son's score of nine was proof that he was fine and that I should not be concerned.

Brady has recently celebrated his ninth birthday. He has his purple belt in karate and loves to snowboard. Brady is home-schooled and in fourth grade. He has brought so much joy to our lives that I can't imagine what life would be without him.

Michael and I have never been able to conceive another child and we are grateful for the gift of our son. I have had a perfectly normal menstrual cycle since Brady's birth.

I think of women who rely on the results of the triple blood screen tests and trust their doctor's advice to consider aborting their baby. They don't realise they could abort a perfectly healthy baby. So many of my friends, and their friends and family have had one of their friends receive the same news from the triple screen test and also have children without the abnormalities predicted by the test.

I hope everyone who reads my story will be inspired to go the extra mile and do their own research. Seek out professionals from whom you can obtain a second opinion. Most of all, go with your gut instincts. You really do know what is best for you, whether you realise it or not. Don't fight your instincts; they could save your life and maybe that of your child!

Jo Litwinowicz

Jo Litwinowicz lives in Cambridgeshire, England. She and her husband became parents in the face of considerable attitudinal and practical barriers. Looking back, Jo has found great joy in raising her son and feels a sense of achievement knowing she proved the doubters wrong.

From 'In My Mind's Eye 1' and 'In My Mind's Eye 2' by Jo Litwinowicz in M. Wates & R. Jade (Eds.). (1999). *Bigger than the sky: Disabled women on parenting*, London: The Women's Press; London. Reprinted with permission.

Jo Litwinowicz

THEY TOLD ME MY CHILD
WOULD WANT A NEW MOTHER

Ever since I can remember, I've dreamt of being married and having at least six children. I was born with cerebral palsy, which makes my right hand and leg do involuntary movements. My speech was very hard to understand until I had a brain operation at the age of 16, which I think has made it easier. As a child I spent more time in hospital than at home, so in some ways I felt more at ease in hospital. Also, my younger brother didn't get picked on so much when I was away.

When I was 22 I decided that I didn't want to go through life 'holding mummy's apron strings', so I went to live in a village especially equipped so that disabled and able-bodied people could live and work together. A couple of years later I met my husband, who lived in the same hostel. He is much older than me and came to the village as a tuberculosis patient, which left him with a very weak chest and one lung.

About three months before our wedding I made an appointment to talk to the doctor about going on the pill. Even though my husband and I both loved children, we thought it would be wrong to bring a child into the world if that child was going to suffer because I couldn't do things like other mums and my husband couldn't run around like other dads. But deep down I still hoped we would have a child.

The doctor told us that as my husband was on all kinds of medication he didn't think he would be able to father a child, and it was unlikely that I could have children, but he'd make an appointment for us to see the family planning clinic. He said the pill would be unsuitable for me and told us not to worry about contraception for the moment. We got an appointment to see the family planning clinic, but it was fourteen weeks after our wedding so, even though our doctor had told us not to bother, we still took our own precautions.

As the date for the appointment grew nearer, I was beginning to panic. Secretly I wanted to get pregnant and felt as if I was waving goodbye to my dream. I also felt really rough and thought I had food poisoning. After another week, I still hadn't shaken it off so I went to see the doctor. Our doctor was on holiday, so I saw his partner who asked me if I could be pregnant. I said that I didn't think so. Still, he took my sample and told me to come back on Friday for the result. I didn't tell my husband about the test as I didn't want him to get excited unnecessarily. On the Friday I woke up feeling dizzy and ill. As my husband worked opposite the surgery I asked him to get the result of a test I had done. I told him to go in at 11 am and if the receptionist said that it was negative then he should go back to work, but if it was positive, I wanted him to come straight home.

By 11:30 he hadn't come back, so I decided I couldn't be pregnant, which I had suspected all along, but I still felt disappointed. When he came home at 12:30 I was preparing dinner. I was facing the hob and I didn't dare to look at him. I said, 'Did you remember to go to the surgery for me?' He didn't answer so I turned around and there was a wide grin on his face. 'Hello, little mum' he said.

When he had gone to the surgery, the doctor had come out of his room and shook his hand saying, 'Congratulations, how do you feel, being a dad-to-be?' When he recovered from the shock, my husband went back to work and told his mates. On the way home he met some of my friends and told them the great news and they said that I must be over the moon, at which point my husband said, 'Oh God, I forgot to tell my own wife she's expecting!' Still in this house we do things differently.

When the news had sunk in, my husband and I sat down and had a serious talk. We knew it was going to be an uphill struggle to convince the authorities that we could manage, and we knew that they would put obstacles in our way. We had already talked about all the pitfalls in caring for a child and we wanted this child so much, but the biggest step was getting the doctors, social workers and everyone else on our side. We wanted them to understand that we were going into this with our eyes wide open. Once we'd achieved that, half the battle would be won.

By Sunday we had got used to the fact that we were going to become parents, so we went down to the phone box to ring my mum and dad. I said to mum, 'How would you like to be a gran?' There was silence for what seemed an eternity. I heard mum calling dad to the phone and she asked me to repeat what I had said so I told them that I was expecting. Their reaction devastated me. 'Well Jo, that news has turned this day into a tragic day. You are an irresponsible and stupid girl.' They might as well have kicked me in the stomach; I was so upset that I slammed the phone down. If my parents' reaction was bad, what chance did we have with complete strangers?

When I went to see my doctor at his antenatal clinic his first words were, 'God, you were the last person I thought I'd see down here.' 'Sorry to disappoint you,' I replied. He asked how we felt about the prospect of becoming parents, and we told him that deep down we had both secretly pined for a child and it was the greatest news ever. His response was to say that throughout my pregnancy, if ever I wanted an abortion, he could arrange it. I was totally horrified and said it would *never* be an option, even if they found there was something wrong with the baby. We were disabled and could cope with a disabled child. Didn't he think we should have a choice? Didn't he think we were capable of *thinking for ourselves*? Just because I'm in a wheelchair and can't use my limbs properly it shouldn't automatically exclude me from the happiness of having a child of my own.

I was so livid with the doctor. He said, 'You can get off the soapbox now, but please go ahead and think about what I said,' so I replied, 'If *you'll* think about what *I* said.'

The next day there was a knock at the door and this woman said she was from Family Planning and could she come in for a chat. I joked, 'You're a bit too late.' She went on, saying how hard it was going to be to raise a child, and told me that I couldn't possibly manage in my condition. I said, 'What condition? You don't know me and what I'm capable of. For your information I'll manage like any mother. Nobody knows how to bring up a child until it's there. Everyone's different and I will have different problems and I'll be ready for them when they crop up and I'll solve them like any other parent.' She said, 'Well, you wouldn't consider an abortion then?' I said, 'NO WAY!'

She calmly went on, 'You do realise that when your child can walk and talk it will come to you and say, "I hate you, mother, because you can't talk properly, you dribble and you're in a wheelchair and I want a new mother."' I began to see red and if my husband hadn't come in, I dread to think what I'd have done to that woman! He opened the door wide and explained that he had heard what was said. 'For your information, we WANT THIS BABY. Get out of our home and don't come upsetting my wife, except to apologise, but do make an appointment first. If you were so concerned that we couldn't look after a child, why didn't you come and see us sooner, before we got married?' She said, 'I was very busy,' and my husband remarked, 'Not too busy to rush down here to tell us to get rid of our baby.' I was in a terrible state.

The doctor came to see us about three hours later. He said, 'What have you been up to, upsetting all the professional people now!' We told him our version and he was most apologetic. We spent two hours discussing the situation and how we felt. We really thrashed it out and then the doctor said, 'Well, you've thought it through and you've convinced me. From now on I'll do everything in my power to help you.' I cried with joy that we actually had our doctor on side at last. True to his word, he was a tower of strength for us and will always be a dear friend.

On New Year's Day I went into hospital for what I thought would be a fortnight but I ended up staying there until my child was born, four months later. The consultant told me I had very high blood pressure and said he would like to keep me in hospital for at least a fortnight so they could run some tests. He assured me that there was nothing to worry about as far as the baby was concerned. Instead of rising, my weight had fallen. I was usually nine stone but now I weighed seven-and-a-half. Every time I ate or drank I got terrible indigestion and had to be sick, and every so often I felt dizzy.

Even though I'd spent half of my life in hospital I felt very nervous this time. The nursing staff weren't at ease handling me at first. I don't think there was much call for helping a severely disabled mum through her pregnancy. I was put in a room on my own. Because I was on a drip and they could only use my good hand for it, I couldn't even read a book. I didn't have a television to lessen the boredom and there wasn't anyone to talk to. The nurses were walking around me as if they were treading on eggshells and I was too frightened to say anything in case it upset the running of the ward. The bed was too high for me to get out of, so I had to use a bedpan, which I hated. I couldn't even look forward to visiting hours because it was impossible for my husband to come during the week. He worked until 5:30 pm and the last bus home was 6 pm. On Sunday the last bus was 2 pm. This meant I could only see my husband once a week, on Saturdays, but we wrote to each other twice a week and it was like courting all over again!

On the fifth day they found a lower bed for me and I was put on the main ward. I soon settled down, the other women got used to me and we chatted endlessly. At the end of the fortnight the consultant said he thought it would be better if I stayed with them until my baby was born so they could monitor us carefully. I knew I would be in the best place if something went wrong, and I was grateful to them for caring, but I regretted not being able to spend this important time with my husband, preparing for the birth of our baby, him missing the first kick and the bonding of the three of us. So every Saturday the nurses made my husband's visit very special and important. They waited for my husband to come before they put the monitor on me to see and hear the baby's heartbeat and I had scans when he was there.

On Monday mornings the consultant and his students always ended up round my bed discussing how my baby was going to be born, as I wanted a natural birth. I didn't want to be put to sleep and miss the big moment. So every week we used to talk about how we were going to do it so as to minimise my spasms.

From about seven and a half months the consultant was getting worried about me and kept saying they should start thinking about inducing the baby, but I kept prolonging it, saying I was okay. But as April came he put his foot down and it was decided that the great day was going to be 24 April, and that I would be awake for it, so I was over the moon.

At 9 pm on Easter Sunday, I had a bath while the nurse prepared the woman opposite me, as they were going to induce her. We were laughing and she kept saying, 'You wait, it'll be your turn in about ten days and I'm coming back to torment you when you deliver.' So I said, 'Like Dick Turpin saying, "Stand and Deliver",' and we all roared with laughter. Even the nurses joined in after a bit. At 10 pm I lay down and found I was wet, even though I had just been to the loo. I told the nurse and she said, 'It's all that laughing. I'll be with you when I finish.' By this time the mattress was absolutely sodden. I couldn't understand it as I was sure I hadn't drunk that much. When the nurse came, she took one look and said, 'Your waters have broken; you're in labour.' I didn't know what to think; it was if a hundred and one things went through my mind in that moment. The ward was cheering and the woman who was going to be induced said, 'It's not fair; *I* went through all that preparation for tomorrow and *you* go into labour!'

My consultant was away on holiday so his standby came to see me at 11 pm. He knew that I wanted to be awake but he said that this was very unexpected, they weren't at full staff and it was the middle of the night, so there was no alternative but to put me to sleep. I was disappointed but on the other hand I wanted the baby to arrive, so I didn't mind. I was told they'd be ready for me about 2 am. Meanwhile, a nurse phoned my friend to see if my husband could come down.

My son was born on Easter Monday at 2:45 am, and weighed 6 lb 6 oz. The nurse brought him out for my husband to hold, so he was the first to see him. I would love to have seen my husband's face when he held the baby. I remember waking up in a ward with my husband standing by the bed and asking him what we had.

When I saw my son, the tears streamed down my face; it was the greatest moment of my life. But after a while, when he was feeding, I suddenly had this strange sensation that I didn't have any maternal feeling towards him. I knew that I loved this baby, but it wasn't real love; it was a weird feeling and I can't find the right words to express it. I didn't dare tell anyone how I was feeling, in case they took my son away. I didn't even tell my husband, so it just stayed bottled inside me.

At 9 am the ward sister asked me how I was, and I said I was a bit woozy. She said they were going to put me in the corner of the ward next to the nursery so that I would have room to move up in my wheelchair when I eventually got up. So I was moved and the curtains were pulled round me. At the time I didn't mind as all I did was sleep. After the third day I felt better so I asked the nurses if I could have the curtains drawn back, but I was told it would be better to leave the curtains as they were for the time being. I felt very upset and isolated as I saw the mums pushing their babies back and forward to the nursery and talking to each other.

When my son, who we named Peter, cried, I had to rely on the nurses to get him or change him as the crib moved around on wheels and it was dangerous for me to try on my own. At feeding times the nurse used to come and plonk Peter in my arms, attach him to the breast, leave me for 15 minutes and then rush back to change sides. I was okay with the baby on my left side but I needed help with the right. The nurses were, as usual, short staffed. My right arm made involuntary movements so my son was going up and down while I was feeding him. He looked highly uncomfortable and I wasn't at ease doing it. When I asked for help, it was always, 'In a minute,' which turned out to be at least 20. I used to cuddle my son and tell him how we'd be going home soon and things would be okay. In my mind's eye I had sorted out how I was going to cope with breastfeeding Peter and doing things for him once we were home. Here he was waking every two hours wanting a feed but we would have to wait another two hours, which wasn't fair. If a nurse came by I would get her to lift Peter out for me so that I could cuddle him. I would give him a crafty little feed on the left side but I was panicking in case a nurse came and caught me.

On the fourth day I asked if I could have a shower and go to the loo. A nurse came with me as it was my first time out of bed since Peter was born. My wheelchair couldn't fit into the bathroom because the doors were too narrow, so I suggested that I use the shower and loo down at the antenatal ward, but I was told firmly, 'No'. They said I would have to keep having bedpans and bedbaths, which made me feel twice as powerless as I was feeling already.

Anyway, one morning Peter was screaming his head off as his feed was due at 10 am and by 10:20 nobody had come. I felt Peter and he was drenched. I'd had enough of waiting, so I knelt on my bed and drew the crib as close as I could, then put my left hand under Peter and started to lift him out. Suddenly the crib moved away and I was left outstretched over the bed still holding Peter in the crib. I was like that for ten minutes before a nurse appeared and then I was told off as if I were a child. I found quite a number of nurses on the ward treated me as if I was simple, which aggravated me, but I had to bite my tongue for my baby's sake, as I needed their help and support.

On the seventh day my consultant returned from his Easter break and said, 'I told you to wait for me.' I said that I wished I had, and began to tell him how I felt about everything. He was so cross that the curtains had been pulled around me all the time. The nurse dug out a crib without wheels that I could use, which was much better, and the curtains were drawn back so at least I could see and talk to the other mums. I was beginning to feel human again, but I was still eager to go home, as the longer I stayed, the more the courage that I had built up for coping with Peter at home slowly ebbed away.

That night some new night staff came. They were very nice and the nurse told me that I should breastfeed my son whichever way I felt comfortable. She showed me how I could feed Peter properly on the right side so that we were both relaxed. We tucked Peter in tightly with me while I lay on the right side letting my breast flop just above his face so he could easily latch onto it himself when he wanted to, and let go of it if he needed a rest. This is how I was planning to feed Peter when I got him home. But the day staff didn't want me to feed Peter with him lying beside me, so I had to continue as before until I could go home, which couldn't come quick enough for me.

On the tenth day I had my stitches out. I said to the nurse, 'That means I can go home now,' as I had seen mums who had their stitches out go home within an hour. Fifteen minutes later the sister came to me and said, 'We've just been talking about you. We realise you're eager to go home but we think it would be wiser if you stayed with us until your son is about ten weeks old. We'll bring his own cot from home, and some other things, so you can show us if you can manage, as we've been doing everything for you so far.' I told her that everything was out of my reach here, plus I wasn't allowed to feed Peter the way I wanted to, plus I found things uncomfortable, and I would like to go home that evening when my husband and friend came.

She said they weren't ready to discharge me, so I said, 'I'm sorry, but if I don't go tonight I will lose all my courage to cope with Peter at home.' So I had to sign my own discharge forms.

The consultant came to say cheerio, which was nice of him, and I felt that he understood my decision. He gave me an appointment to see him with Peter six weeks later. Then at 7 pm my friend and husband took me home.

Postcript

Jo's husband died six years ago. Last year she suffered a heart attack and a stroke. Although life has been an uphill struggle, she takes great pride in her son Peter, who is now 25 and works as a chef. He tells her he is 'so glad to be her son' and that he 'appreciates life even more' because of her. She writes: 'When he says this to me I feel like crying. I wish I could meet all the medical people and cynics who told me that I wouldn't be able to bring a child up and that when the child can talk he will come to me and say, 'I don't like a mum in a wheelchair.' I wish I could see their faces now. Many people told me Peter wouldn't be good at anything. He has now bought his own house, has a girlfriend and is doing a job he loves.

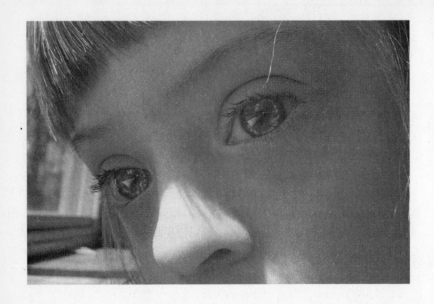

Michelle Harmon

Michelle and her childhood sweetheart Jim live at the base of a mountain in Maine, USA, with their three children, two dogs and two cats.

Michelle Harmon

THE MOST BEAUTIFUL FACE ON EARTH

I am a 33-year-old Mom from Maine. I had a daughter in January 1989. Her dad walked out on me when I was pregnant, telling me to get an abortion or get out of his life. I was terrified – I almost considered it. I was very lucky I found a place that cared for me. They gave me a little pair of knitted booties, baby blue, something tangible to hold onto while awaiting the birth of this very unplanned child. Her dad did leave, and has never seen her. My fiancé Jim has raised her and been her true father. It was a trying time, but I think it was preparation for the future.

As it turned out, having Kristin was the easy part. For seven years after her birth, Jim and I tried to have another baby. It just wasn't happening. I started college, determined to make up for the rotten childhood I'd had. My daughter was the entire focus of our lives. It seemed she would be the one and only.

Months after starting college, I discovered, much to my happiness, that I was pregnant! I had gut-wrenching morning sickness, but happily put up with whatever it took to have my beautiful son. He was born in September 1995, blonde and curly and fair. We named him Jesse, and he filled a hole we hadn't known we had. We settled into life, thinking our world was complete.

When Jesse was about a year old, we got a call. Our little nephew, Alex, was in a foster home and needed a place to call his own. We applied for our foster license, and when he was eight months old, the day before Jim's birthday, we brought Alex home. He would become our second son. He was a sweet-natured, beautiful baby. But within days, at his first pediatric check-up, he was diagnosed with cerebral palsy. I thought, 'I can handle that,' and so we moved forward yet again, a little bigger, a few more appointments, but happy nonetheless.

When Alex had been here just seven weeks, I discovered I was unexpectedly pregnant again. It was quite a shock, from one to four children in about a year-and-a-half. Our daughter Kristin was learning to share our time and attention in a big way. Again, we said, 'We can handle it', and moved forward. We had great hopes that the new baby would be a girl; two of each sounded perfect to us who had thought we would never have more than one.

My best friend from elementary school had had a child with Down syndrome. I never believed it could happen to us. I was wrong. I was sitting in a hospital room with Jesse, who had been admitted the day after Alex had left the hospital for the very same thing – rotovirus – when I got a message from home to call my doctor. I was exhausted. I had been a week in hospital already, and facing yet another stay with my very sick little boy.

I called the doctor, expecting a reminder that in all the craziness of my schedule lately, I had missed an appointment. He informed me that my AFP test had come back indicative of Down syndrome. I was shocked to hear the words. They asked me to come to do a level II ultrasound to look for markers that would give us a better idea. Jim and I arranged for someone to stay with the kids, and up we went, expecting this huge mistake to be clarified and to go home to our growing brood happily free of this new worry. We couldn't fathom the thought that we would have a disabled child.

The doctor did a very in-depth exam. He looked for all the markers that might indicate Down syndrome. I remember lying on that table, laughing as we saw her tiny fingers on the ultrasound. All the doctor could find were shortened femur bones.

I looked to the side of the bed at her daddy and giggled. His legs were pretty short, too. We talked for a moment about French Canadians and their notoriously short legs. We were begging to hear the words that would exempt us from further testing. Something to blame the AFP results on – anything but Down syndrome.

There were no other markers. As sure as we were of our date of conception, we convinced ourselves that it was a simple miscalculation. But the doctor wanted to do an amniocentesis right away. We knew that no matter what it said, we wouldn't abort. We drove home that afternoon giggling about Jim's short legs, comparing notes on the beautiful child we had just spent several hours getting a preview of.

And so, we went on with the business of raising the kids, and adding on to our house in preparation for the new baby. We now knew it was a little girl. We imagined her a towhead [redhead] with blue eyes and curly hair, a healthy 'normal' addition to our family.

On 27 June 1998, I went into labour very suddenly at home. I told Jim, who was working on the addition for the baby's room. We figured we had a while before we had to start the 25-minute drive to the hospital. There was no film in the camera, so I told Jim we should go shopping first. We couldn't know it then, but we were spending our last hours as the Jim and Michelle we had been up until that day. By the end of the day, we would become different versions of ourselves, affected forever by the overwhelming love we would come to feel for our incredibly special little girl.

We stopped by Radio Shack. I stayed in the car while he ran in to get the film, then on to buy a new nightgown. As I browsed the racks, the pains started coming hard and fast. We hurried out of the store and to the hospital. Jim walked me upstairs and settled me in, then went to park the car. By the time he returned, I was in hard labour. Twelve minutes after getting to the hospital, our baby girl was born – 6 lbs 7 oz and not breathing real well.

They took her to the warming table and started working on her. I wasn't terribly concerned; I could hear her breathing. But as the minutes ticked by and they continued to work on her, I felt this absolute certainty that there was something very different about this baby. After what seemed an eternity, they finally brought her over to show me. They laid her on my stomach, and she raised her head. The very second she looked at me, I knew.

I can remember that moment with a clarity like none I have ever experienced. In a split second I realised that the very thing I had been so afraid of was the thing that would become most precious to me. 'Down syndrome' was just a phrase, and this was my child. I asked, 'What are the chances this baby has Down syndrome?' They all acted like they were shocked that I would ask the question, until I reminded them of the AFP and Dr Bowley.

She was whisked away immediately. All the nurses kept telling me not to worry, she was fine. They all thought she didn't have Down syndrome; she had none of the usual features, except the slanted eyes. I saw them checking and rechecking the palms of her hands for the typical single crease which indicates the condition.

I knew, though. I knew from the minute I saw her. And what once would have devastated me somehow changed me. This was *my* baby, not some 'retarded child' I was seeing on TV. The things I had thought about my friend's baby came back to haunt me then. I was not anguished about my child with Down syndrome, but about the many children with Down syndrome who had mysteriously come through my life prior to her, small messengers whose presence I had never acknowledged. I was ashamed. I loved this baby without reservation. I knew that I had some making up to do for my friend's child, for never having seen her as the unique and beautiful child she was. I was already learning about my own prejudices.

Nine days later, I took my baby girl home from the hospital. I told everyone who would listen about the Down syndrome. I was so proud of this child, I actually surprised myself. Down syndrome lost its novelty. I still sometimes see these subtle features and think this is most certainly the most beautiful face on earth. My prejudice gets the better of me sometimes – I just can't see anything about Ciarra as a negative. I know my soul is different for having her. I am more open, more spiritual, more in tune with life. My kids adore this baby sister who is almost 4 now. My oldest daughter is 13. I go to her school and I immediately lose the baby to her friends.

Ciarra attends a regular preschool program; she was potty-trained before she was 3, and is a very independent little kid. She is funny and spirited, stubborn and witty. She whistles little songs all day long. She idolises her big brother. She loves to draw, and can put all the details into a drawing of a face.

At 5 years old, this child they told me would be so unworthy of life, such a burden, has defied all predictions. She is in a mainstream kindergarten class where she holds her own nicely and is doing most things like any other child her age. Letters and words seem to be her strength.

She has so many friends that sometimes we get tired of dragging her to playdates and parties. One little boy was allowed to invite three boys and three girls when he turned six. He chose Ciarra. He *chose* her. All those worries I had about kids shying away from her have turned out to be the exact opposite. She is like a magnet. Sometimes the other kids want to baby her, because she is still so tiny, but she lets them know she is not a baby. Her teachers have fallen in love with her. Many of them were afraid of Down syndrome when this whole process started. Now they are like me, grateful for the opportunity to know her. She continues to touch people with her sweetness and surprise them with her ability.

Ciarra is a little girl who has been the best teacher I can ever imagine having. She is joy like no other.

I hope my story helps even one family to think about continuing a pregnancy with a Down syndrome diagnosis. This thing I once so feared, I am so at ease with now. I wouldn't change this little girl if I had the magic pill today. I'm honoured to be her mum. If you are a mum expecting a child with Down syndrome, try to remember that the baby you are carrying today is the same baby you felt moving yesterday, the same baby you loved unconditionally the day before he or she was diagnosed.

I continue to be amazed by the hearts such a small child has touched. She seems to have a way with people that I have never seen before. I wonder if it is her cheerfulness or her simple joy in everything. The optimist in me likes to think it is just Ciarra's magic, and that the lessons she teaches will stay with people. Maybe someday it won't be so scary to have a child with Down syndrome. Maybe someday 95 percent of her peers will not be eliminated. For right now, I can only raise her to be a decent human being and a good friend. I can hope her academic success continues, and that she will change the world.

But in my heart I know that the best changes she has brought are within her own family, within me. I am blessed beyond words by this little girl. That blessing seems to know no end, it grows and grows and fills my heart daily. People may ask if it's hard to have a kid like her. I wish they could know the truth. Sure, there are days I get tired. She asks a lot of questions, and she is in perpetual motion. But I wouldn't trade her for the world. In terms of medical issues, the demons that we were told we would have to hold at bay have all but disappeared. We go for an echocardiogram next week; the hole in her heart is closing up. The physical stuff just isn't an issue. Funny how we were told how dire it would be. In five years, we have learned that doctors just don't know.

Ciarra has changed me so much. I have slowed down to enjoy the world more. She is perpetually hopeful, and most often smiling. She is the closest thing to an angel I will ever see. Through her, I have started an online support group. We are a close-knit community. I try to lend a little hope when I connect with other women shortly after the diagnosis of their child. Ciarra is helping me to make a difference in this world.

Afterword

Genetic screening and abortion:
Ratifying social prejudice through reproductive 'choices'

While the 'old' style eugenics employed coercive means, for the most part the new eugenics advances under the guise of facilitating individual choices – part of the rhetoric of the 'right to choose.' As Ruth Hubbard had already observed in 1987:

> There may be no need for eugenic legislation. Physicians and scientists need merely provide the techniques that make individual women, and parents, responsible for implementing the society's prejudices, so to speak, by choice (in Baruch et al., 1987, p.232).

Laura Hershey agrees with Hubbard's view, suggesting that while prenatal screening may appear to give pregnant women more power, in reality women are asked to ratify social prejudices through their reproductive 'choices'. As she puts it:

> I cannot help thinking that in most cases, when a woman terminates a previously wanted pregnancy expressly to avoid giving birth to a disabled child, she is buying into obsolete assumptions about that child's future. And she is making a statement about the desirability or the relative worth of such a child. Abortion based on disability results from, and in turn strengthens, certain beliefs: children with disabilities (and by implication adults with disabilities) are a burden to family and society: life with a disability is scarcely worth

living; preventing the birth is an act of kindness; women who bear disabled children have failed (Hershey, 1994, pp. 28–29).

Mary Johnson, an American disability activist, also believes decisions are made on the basis of discriminatory cultural assumptions.

> This is . . . a discussion about the thinking that prompts the woman, or the couple, to make certain specific decisions based on cultural assumptions that have been shaped by discriminatory practices and attitudes – against disabled people.
>
> A decision to abort based on the fact that the child is going to have specific individual characteristics such as mental retardation, or in the specific case of cystic fibrosis, a buildup of mucus in the lungs, says that those characteristics take precedence over the living itself. That they are so important and so negative, that they overpower any positive qualities there might be in being alive (Johnson, 1990, p. 14).

Indeed, any 'positive qualities' are undermined and crushed beneath a weight of 'costs-benefit' arguments, perfectionist goals and eugenicist imperatives which require elimination of the imperfect, and a society which resists adjusting to accommodate every (type of) body.

The new genetics and apartheid

In their 2005 book *Disability in Australia: Exposing a Social Apartheid*, Gerard Goggin and Christopher Newell place new genetics, including the Human Genome Project (sorting out 'good genes' from 'bad genes'), embryonic stem cell and cloning research, in the context of apartheid – treating people with disabilities as undesirable, as *other*.[1] They see this response as part of the catastrophising of disability.[2] They write:

For many hundreds of years, people with disabilities have been marked as different, separated and often cast out from society. Those deemed mad, sick, uncontrollable, deaf, blind, mute, leprous, and disfigured have been subject to laws and mores branding them different and a people apart (Goggin and Newell, 2005, p. 123).

Associate Professor of Medical Ethics at the University of Tasmania, Christopher Newell has drawn attention to how the media excitement over embryonic stem cells and the magic cures they might one day supposedly provide, marginalise the needs of people living with disabilities:

Rather than dealing with the human rights of people with disability, all this media hype serves to do is reinforce the notion of disability as a personal tragedy ... the moment that the stem cell decision was made [in Australia] it was as if the answer to disability had been found. Accordingly, disability again disappeared from the nation's agenda, left dormant until the next time powerful interests appropriate it (Newell, 2002, p. 15).

Other disability activists felt the same. Erik Leipoldt and Maurice Corcoran, who both have quadriplegia, said what makes the lives of quadriplegics so difficult was 'inadequate support services, de-humanising institutions, high levels of unemployment and exclusion from regular education' – not restrictions on scientific research (in Cook 2004, p. 28).

Fiona Campbell offers a similar analysis:

John Radford is correct then when he refers to 'disability' as the Enlightenment's 'recidivist element' – signifying an ontology of failure, hopelessness requiring surveillance, repair and management. Hence, 'disablised bodies' throughout Western history have been represented as sub-human organisms, monsters, freaks or as an objects [*sic*] of ridicule, sympathy and burdens of charity (2000, p. 309).[3]

But why bother changing conditions for people with disabilities (in Victoria, Australia, there are 9-year-old children with disabilities living in aged care nursing homes because there is nowhere else for them to go; Ellingsen, 2004) – when we can get rid of them in the first place – *genetically cleanse* our society of them? Mary Johnson argues: 'A disabled fetus represents for parents a problem that may have far more to do with society than with disability. Disabled children confront a hostile environment' (Johnson, 1990, p. 14).

Mr Shahraz Kayani's daughter confronted a hostile environment when she was not allowed to migrate to Australia to join her Australian citizen father – because she had a disability. Kayani, who came to Australia as a refugee, had been unsuccessful in multiple attempts to bring his wife and three daughters from Pakistan to Australia to join him. The application had originally been refused because one of his daughters had cerebral palsy and authorities estimated it would cost taxpayers too much to care for her (even though the family had undertaken to cover all costs associated with her care themselves). The little girl was treated as *other*, to be kept apart from a country that did not want her and to be denied family reunion because of her disability.

In 2001, Mr Kayani poured petrol over himself and set himself alight outside the Federal Parliament in protest against the Government's thwarting of his efforts to reunite his family. He later died from his injuries (in *Sydney Morning Herald*, 29 May 2001, p. 3).

Blaming the individual

We live in a society – especially those of us in the more comfortable west – that fears and despises suffering and doesn't know how to deal with pain and death. People who suffer chronic conditions remind us of our own vulnerabilities. The first tendency is to blame those who suffer as somehow having wrought destruction upon themselves by their own choices; as having disgraced themselves. Gwen Anderson writes (1999, p. 130):

> Suffering is conceived as something detrimental to human existence and incompatible with happiness. This imperative is based on a world-view that defines human suffering as pain that need not be endured, or as punishment, hardship or disaster due to wrongful choices. The belief that genetic conditions are 'defects' that can be avoided perpetuates a myth that leads to personal shame and family disgrace when such an event occurs.[4]

Hence it is not surprising that so many pregnant women, faced with a medical diagnosis that something will be 'wrong' with their child, opt for abortion as the only – and indeed best – solution for all.

Alison Brookes says the lack of appropriate care was sometimes such a concern it could override even strong ethical objections to abortion. She says women in her study 'decried the lack of available community support and access to care that framed their decision-making process regarding reproduction' (Brookes, 2001, p. 137).

Australian Jesuit priest and social commentator, Frank Brennan, picks up on this:

> If the state is to extend equal protection to all citizens, including the most vulnerable . . . The mother of the disabled child, like the mother of the normal child, must have the right to bear her child and to receive assistance from the state with the provision of the basic necessities for the child's wellbeing (Brennan, 2002, p. 7).

However prenatal technologies and genetic engineering further the view that the individual is to blame. Thus the oppression goes unchallenged (Shakespeare, 1999). According to Gregor Wolbring (2004) the prevailing 'Management of "the disability", of the disabled person or person-to-be and the usage of new technologies such as Nanotechnology, Biotechnology, Information technology and cognitive sciences (NBIC) are aimed at "cure" (for example gene therapy, stem cell regenerative medicine, nanomedicine), "prevention" (prenatal genetic and non genetic diagnostics and preimplantation genetic diagnostics with the attached selection method), or "adaptation", of the person by various normalizing assistive devices (e.g. cochlear implants, artificial legs, retina chips, brain machine interfaces) to ensure functioning or existence as normative as possible.'

This 'management of disability', is based on a medical model of disability which according to Wolbring (2004) 'is much too limited to address the needs of disabled people and other marginalized groups, contributing to overall global health inequities and the likelihood that the Millenium Development Goals (MDGs) will not be met. It results in too narrow a policy/research focus that fails to address health as a state of complete physical, mental and social well-being.' It ignores the WHO aim 'to ensure equal opportunities and promotion of human rights for people with disabilities, especially those who are poor' and it ignores that, according to Wolbring, 'Current understanding about what constitutes a disability and what individuals with a disability have to contribute to society has reframed disability as an issue of social entitlement, economic opportunity and human rights, as evidenced by the flurry of progressive legislation and new programs around the world, including a UN international convention to promote and protect the rights of disabled persons.' An attitudinal or ideological shift is required so that able-ism can be seen as on a par with, for example, racism and sexism.

Lisa Blumberg observes:

It says something very telling about our society that we seem to care more about distinguishing between the normal and the 'abnormal' prenatally than we do about creating conditions where all people can lead the best possible lives . . .

Parenting a disabled child will become a more viable option for more people if society provides more support to parents in general (1994b, p. 150).[5]

And Ruth Hubbard emphasises that 'a woman must . . . feel empowered not to terminate . . . [a pregnancy involving a fetus with a disability] confident that the society will do what it can to enable her and her child to live fulfilling lives' (Hubbard, 1997, p. 199).

The erosion of empathy

We must ask the question – where is the true malfunction? During a major abortion debate in the West Australian Parliament in 1998, seven senior doctors, including Professor Fiona Stanley, the Founding Director of the Institute of Child Health Research, sent a letter to State Members of Parliament, warning of the 'implications of curbing access to abortion'. The letter pointed out that 100 of the 9000 terminations in that state every year involved foetal abnormalities. 'Whilst some of these children would die soon after birth, some would survive the disabilities and need services that are already stretched to the limit,' the letter said (Stanley, F. et al., 1998, p. 5).

Phil Grano, coordinator of Villamanta Legal Service, a community-based agency representing the disabled in Victoria, Australia, says that if disabled children become rare, the world will be a less tolerant place – especially if their rarity encouraged a culture of blame against those who receive disability pensions or state support to care for disabled children.

People with disabilities create a connection between people . . . They shatter our small horizons. They open us up to intangible experiences of community. They draw acceptance from us because they are just who they are, without pretence. The nature of day-to-day life for people with disabilities is hard, but I haven't met many who don't want to live. They are tenacious about life (in Toy and Milburn, 2000, p. 3).

Commentators like Richard Titmuss (1970) and Hans S. Reinders (2000) argue that sympathy and altruism are developed through the care of vulnerable groups – that opportunities for the expression of altruism result in more caring behaviour. Therefore a culture of screening and abortion limiting the numbers of those with disabilities, erodes our sense of caring and possibly paves the way for less tolerance and acceptance of difference.[6] As Reinders observes:

It has been reported that parents of disabled children sometimes describe the success of parenting these children in terms of a 'transformation experience'. Only when they were ready to let this child change their lives, including their views of themselves, were they able to enter into a process of learning and sharing . . . it suggests that it takes a particular kind of people to care for disabled persons and to enable them to flourish . . . the future of disabled people in our society will in large part depend on whether or not there will be such people . . . the crucial questions then becomes how liberal society can produce the kind of people who are willing to have themselves transformed by what their society portrays and evaluates as defective children (Reinders, 2000, p. 177).

An example of such a child providing his or her parents with a transformative experience appeared in the Letters section of *The Age* (Melbourne, Australia), in July 2000 (p. 16), titled 'I wouldn't give him up for the world' by Karen Dymke:

At 32 weeks into my pregnancy I learnt via an ultra-sound that my son had a significant brain abnormality. To put it simply, he had half of his brain missing. It was a terrible shock. The outlook appeared very grim. My son was born at term and presents with a number of difficulties. He has a shunt to drain fluid from his brain, has mild cerebral palsy and has some speech difficulties. He is now almost 10 years old. He is also a fantastic kid and an inspiration to everyone who knows him. It hasn't always been easy. But what a gift he has been to us! I wouldn't give him up for the world. Not then, not ever.

Louise Drinkwater also gives expression to this transformative experience, speaking about her daughter Molly, who has Down syndrome.

She's an incredibly happy little girl. She lights up our lives . . . I've been a person who thought academic achievement was really important, and it's been a beautiful learning experience to realise that value is about the soul of the person. Molly has really helped me to sit back and enjoy the moment rather than racing to get ahead (in Robotham and Smith, 2004).

And Lise Poirier-Groulx writes in this book:

Although the journey has been incredibly difficult for the entire family, we have absolutely no regrets. The blessings which accompanied this little one into our lives far outweigh the sorrows we have experienced. We have grown and learned so very much through him. Every day, we witness how he touches people's hearts, and people's lives are changed just because of who he is. Everyone who knows him loves him!

Losing our humanity

In his 1999 article 'The Moral Meaning of Genetic Technology', Leon Kass warns of the view that individuals are 'mere raw material for manipulation and homogenization' (Kass, 1999, p. 38). Con-

trolling the product can only be achieved through deperson-
alisation. As he puts it (p. 37):

> . . . the conquest of disease, aggression, pain, anxiety, suffering,
> and grief unavoidably comes at the price of homogenization,
> mediocrity, pacification, trivialized attachments, debasement of
> taste, and souls without love or longing.

We may become so dehumanised, we won't even recognise that
in the quest to be perfect, we are no longer even human. Kass says
we must act quickly to 'defend the increasingly beleaguered vestiges
and principles of our human dignity' (Kass, 1999, p. 38). Francis
Fukuyama writes of what he calls Factor X, or human essence,
which 'unites all human beings', and gives us 'dignity and moral
status.'

> What is it that we want to protect from any future advances in
> biotechnology? The answer is, we want to protect the full range of
> our complex, evolved natures against attempts at self-modification.
> We do not want to disrupt either the unity or the continuity of
> human nature, and thereby the human rights that are based on it'
> (Fukuyama, 2002, pp. 153, 171, 172).

Bioethicist George Annas (1993), writing of the Human
Genome Project, is also concerned about the loss of what it means
to be human. He describes '[B]reaking "human beings" down into
6 billion "parts" as "the ultimate in reductionism."' Annas continues: '. . . what variation will society view as permissible before
an individual's genome is labelled substandard or abnormal? And
what impact would such a construct of genetic normalcy have on
society and on substandard individuals?'

On the Human Genome Project, Martin Rothblatt observes:

> When certain genomes are not allowed to exist, demographic death
> will occur. A trunk of human life will become extinct, its unique

genomic contribution forever lost. Worse still, persons still living with the proscribed genomic characteristic will be seriously devalued – not even deemed worthy of reproduction – often leading to a loss of their civil rights (Rothblatt, 1997, p. 8).

While not directly addressing the subject of this book in her 2004 Sydney Peace Prize lecture, the words of award winning Indian writer and human rights activist Arundhati Roy are none-theless relevant here:

> The assault on vulnerable, fragile sections of society is at once so complete, so cruel and so clever – all encompassing and yet specifically targeted, blatantly brutal and yet unbelievably insidious – that its sheer audacity has eroded our definition of justice (Roy, 2004).

We could be on our way to creating a world of people which fit the title of an article by Tom Wolfe 'Sorry, but Your Soul Just Died' (1996).

Mutual interdependence

Susan Wendell provides a timely reminder of our interde-pendence. Having acquired a disability, she 'began to experience the world as structured for people who have no weaknesses' (1992, p. 63).

> I hope that disabled and able-bodied feminists will join in questioning our cultural obsession with independence and ultimately replacing it with such a model of reciprocity. If *all* the disabled are to be fully integrated into society without symbolizing failure, then we have to change social values to recognize the value of depending on others and being depended upon (Wendell, 1992, p. 76).

Troy Duster, in *Backdoor to Eugenics*, has asked if something labelled a 'defect' is more likely 'an arbitrary social assessment of aesthetics and or potential dependency' (Duster, 1990, p. 4). Jennifer Fitzgerald, in an article titled 'Geneticizing Disability', also observes how a society which worships independence has problems dealing with dependency: 'The power/knowledge structure is being used by society as justification for the removal of a minority group on the basis that unproductiveness and dependency are unacceptable characteristics,' she writes (Field, 1996 in Fitzgerald, 1997).

In *For Common Things: Irony, Trust and Commitment in America Today*, Jedediah Purdy discusses the defining moral danger of genetic engineering as fraying our 'sense of common humanity.' In his words:

> What care we take for other people, especially but by no means only those outside our immediate circle of love, is caught up with a sense that we share a common vulnerability . . . At our best we are affected by what Jan Patocka, a Czech philosopher and dissident who died after a beating by the Czechoslovak secret police, used to call 'the solidarity of the shaken': the cleaving together of those who recognize how easily they can be riven apart from one another, from what they value most, and even from their lives . . .
>
> The more we can select against these inconvenient fellow citizens, the more likely we are to grow callous in our treatment of them.
>
> . . . By inviting this confusion, biotechnology has the power to foster the worst kind of indifference. The conviction that our own desires are the world's compass points is among the greatest barriers to genuine respect for other individuals. The more able we become to treat others as vehicles for our own aims, the less readily we conceive of them as intrinsically important (Purdy, 1999, pp. 175, 177, 179).

The women in this book have confronted these impersonal technologies of quality control. Demonstrating remarkable bravery, they have refused to allow themselves or their children to be categorised as genetically disfavoured, to be denied living because they are seen by some as at the bottom of some utilitarian genetically-constructed hierarchy, the subjects of medicalised bigotry,[7] to be fixed and mastered in their life decisions by an ideology of perfectionism and faultlessness.

It is my hope that their examples may provide courage for other women to follow them on their path and demand an end to society's loathing and hatred of anything that is 'other' than fitting in rigidly constructed categories of what constitutes 'normal.' Humanity will be the richer for their resistance. In fact, it depends upon it.

Notes

The new genetics and apartheid

1. An interesting commentary by the Acting Disability Discrimination Commissioner, Dr Sev Ozdowski, on employment issues for people with disabilities, which includes pertinent observations on the under-investment in people with disabilities as employees, can be found at http://www.hreoc.gov.au/disability_rights/speeches/ 2004/aig.htm

2. The catastrophising and pathologising of disability is challenged by Anthony Bartl in The million-dollar question: Why Eastwood's baby got it wrong (2005, p. 21). An arts student at La Trobe University, Bartl suffered C1-C2 complete quadriplegia in a car accident – the same disability that leads to the euthanising of Maggie Fitzgerald (Hilary Swank) in Clint Eastwood's film *Million Dollar Baby*.

    Also commenting on the impact of the film on people with disabilities was Lawrence Carter-Long, member of the board of the Centre for Independence of the Disabled in New York, who wrote:

    > Eastwood and his film's liberal supporters have somehow failed to see – and perhaps worse yet, failed to examine – why disabled people would be hurt and offended. Is the notion of preferring to die rather than choosing to live with a disability so commonplace it merits no reflection by able-bodied movie directors, film critics and audiences? Moreover, are the feelings of real, live disabled people so irrelevant in our culture they aren't even considered when

movies such as *Million Dollar Baby* are made? . . . [The film] plays more to the largely irrational fears of what having a disability might be like rather than the reality of living one's life with a disability . . . (Carter-Long, 2005, p. 12).

Not listening to the voices of the disabled was starkly illustrated in the case of the American woman, Terri Schiavo, whose feeding tube was removed in 2005 to allow death by dehydration. President of Not Dead Yet, Diana Coleman pointed out that 26 national disability organisations took the position that Ms Schiavo should receive food and water but their stance was 'consistently ignored by most of the press, as well as the courts'. See Testimony Before the Subcommittee on Criminal Justice, Drug Policy and Human Resources Of the Committee on Government Reform Of the US House of Representatives Oversight Hearing on "Federal Health Programs and Those Who Cannot Care for Themselves: What Are Their Rights, And Our Responsibilities?" April 19, 2005. See also Nat Hentoff, Terri Schiavo: Judicial Murder, 2005.

3. Campbell, F. (2000). Campbell cites Radford, J. (1994). Intellectual disability and the heritage of modernity. In M. Rioux, & M. Bach (Eds.), *Disability is not measles: New research paradigms in disability* (pp. 9–27).

Blaming the individual

4. Anderson, G. (1999). Nondirectiveness in prenatal genetics: Patients read between the lines. Personal shame and family disgrace are what drove the mother of the previously mentioned baby with suspected dwarfism to seek an abortion. She was overwhelmed by a sense of shame for being pregnant with a child with a disability. In her culture, it was 'bad karma' to give birth to such a child – she was being punished for her sin (see Tankard Reist 2004a). No amount of hand wringing will bring back dead babies after abortion.

5. Blumberg suggests family-strengthening initiatives such as parental leave, part-time and flex-time work, expanded child care alternatives, comprehensive health care programs and programs assisting low income families.

The erosion of empathy

6. See Titmuss, R. M. (1970). *The gift relationship: From human blood to social policy*, and Reinders, H. S. (2000). *The Future of the disabled in liberal society: An ethical analysis.*

Mutual interdependence

7. 'Medicalised bigotry' is Martin Rothblatt's phrase. Rothblatt, M. (1997). *Unzipped genes: Taking charge of baby-making in the new millennium.*

Glossary

Alpha-fetoprotein (AFP) test: A blood test that is performed during pregnancy. This screening test measures the level of AFP in the pregnant woman's blood and indicates the probability that the foetus has one of several birth defects. The AFP level can also be determined using a sample of amniotic fluid. This screening test cannot diagnose a specific condition; it only indicates the increase of risk.

Amniocentesis: A diagnostic procedure performed by inserting a hollow needle through the abdominal wall into the uterus and withdrawing a small amount of fluid from the sac surrounding the foetus. DNA analysis is then performed on the fluid. The test can detect chromosomal disorders such as Down syndrome, or structural defects such as spina bifida, anencephaly, and other inherited metabolic disorders. Later on in a pregnancy, amniocentesis may be used to identify suspected problems such as Rh incompatibility or infection. There is a chance of infection or injury to the foetus, and a chance of miscarriage.

Anencephaly: A neural tube defect where the top of the spinal column fails to close and the brain is incomplete or missing.

Antenatal: The period of pregnancy before birth.

Antenatal care: The usual care given to pregnant women. This may include pre-conception counselling, assessment of risk factors (including maternal health), assessment of foetal well-being and complications, education about normal experiences of pregnancy, emotional aspects (including post-natal depression), antenatal classes, reducing risk of SIDS, parenting issues (including child-proofing the house and coping with crying infants) and birthing care options.

APGAR test: A scoring system for the health status of newborn babies, which includes assessment of heart rate, respiratory effort, muscle tone, reflexes, and skin colour. A score of seven or higher (out of ten) is considered normal. The test is done at one minute after birth and again at five minutes.

Biobanks: Collections of human biological material that may include DNA, cells, tissues or organs. Collection may occur in the context of surgery, medical testing or autopsy within the health care system and the medical sciences. Material may be used for medical, scientific, therapeutic or educational purposes. Biobanks may be privately or publicly funded.

Carcinogenesis: A carcinogen is a substance that causes or is believed to cause cancer. A carcinogenic material is one that is known to cause cancer. The process of forming cancer cells from normal cells or carcinomas is called carcinogenesis.

Cerebral Palsy (CP): A group of disorders which involve loss of movement or loss of other nerve functions. These disorders are caused by injuries to the brain that occur during foetal development or near the time of birth, which can result in the loss of nerve functions in a variety of areas. The typical finding of CP is spasticity (increased muscle tone) which may affect a single limb, one side of the body (spastic hemiplegia), both legs (spastic diplegia) or both arms and legs (spastic quadriplegia). In addition, there may be partial or full loss of movement (paralysis), sensory abnormalities, hearing and vision impairment, speech abnormalities and seizures. Intellectual function may range from extremely bright to severe mental retardation. Cerebral palsy is a non-progressive type of encephalopathy (injury to the brain) and symptoms directly resulting from the disease do not become worse over time. A person with the disorder may improve during childhood if they receive appropriate care from specialists. Some people will need to stay under the immediate care of another person for their entire lives, while others have a case mild enough to pursue fully independent lives.

Chorionic villous sampling (CVS): Prenatal diagnosis procedure where a small part of the placenta (chorionic villi) are removed.

Choroid plexus cysts: Fluid-filled spaces in the choroid plexus (specialised areas in the roof of the brain ventricles that produce the cerebrospinal fluid). They are seen in about 1 percent of all second trimester ultrasounds. Choroid plexus cysts may be seen in one or both sides of the brain. The number, size, and shape of the cysts may vary. Choroid plexus cysts are also found in healthy children and adults.

Chromosomes: Tightly coiled DNA. The visible structures within each cell that house the genes. There are 46 human chromosomes: 22 pairs and 2 sex chromosomes; two X chromosomes for females, one X and one Y chromosome for males. Humans inherit 22 chromosomes plus one sex chromosome from each parent.

Cleft palate or 'hare lip': Congenital (present from before birth) abnormalities that affect the upper lip and the hard and soft palate of the mouth. Severity of the abnormalities may range from a small notch in the lip to a complete fissure (groove) extending into the roof of the mouth and nose. These features can occur separately or together. Cleft lip and palate may occur in association with other syndromes or birth defects. There are numerous causes for these, including mutant genes inherited from one or both parents, and teratogens (drugs, viruses, or other toxins that can cause abnormalities in a developing foetus). These abnormalities can cause feeding difficulties, problems with speech development, and ear infections. A cleft palate is usually closed within the first year of life to enhance normal speech development. Until surgery, a prosthetic device is often fitted over the palate for feeding. Although treatment may extend over several years and require several surgeries depending upon the involvement, most children affected by this disorder can achieve normal appearance, speech, and eating. For some, speech problems may continue.

Cloning: The replication of genetic material, specifically DNA. Individual strands of DNA can be cloned and individual cells can be cloned. Cloning usually applies to replication of all of the genetic material of an organism by transfer of the nucleus of an adult cell into an egg cell from which the nucleus has been removed. The cloned cell can develop as an embryo, be implanted in the uterus of the species cloned and possibly be born, or be destroyed to yield its stem cells for research, possible therapy or other purposes.

Cystic Fibrosis: An inherited disease that affects chloride channels in the body, causing breathing and digestive problems. It affects the mucus and sweat glands of the body and is caused by a defective gene. Thick mucus is formed in the breathing passages of the lungs so that the person is prone to chronic lung infections. Many pancreatic enzymes are blocked from reaching the intestine, causing malabsorption (inadequate absorption of nutrients from the intestinal tract) and malnutrition. Early diagnosis and a comprehensive, multidisciplinary treatment program can lengthen survival time and improve quality of life, and specialty clinics for cystic fibrosis can be found in many communities. Around 40 percent of children with cystic fibrosis live beyond age 18 and the average life span for those who live to adulthood is now 35 years, a dramatic increase over the last three decades. Death is usually caused by lung complications.

DNA: Acronym for DeoxyriboNucleic Acid, the molecule which contains the genetic code. DNA is arranged in the form of a double helix, and the two helices are held together by bonds between the bases Cytosine, Guanine, Thymine and Adenine. The sequence of these bases is the genetic code, usually simplified to combinations of C, G, T, and A.

Down syndrome (also known as trisomy 21): Down syndrome is a chromosome abnormality due to an extra copy of the chromosome 21. This syndrome usually, although not always, results in mental retardation and other conditions. Individuals with Down syndrome have a widely recognised characteristic appearance. Retardation of normal growth and development is typical and most affected children never reach average adult height. Congenital heart defects are sometimes present, and some may require surgical correction. The potential for visual problems, hearing loss, and increased susceptibility to infection mean that children will require screening and treatment at appropriate intervals. The normal life span is shortened by congenital heart disease and an increased incidence of acute leukaemia. Mental retardation is variable, although usually of moderate severity.

Dwarfism (technical names: Panhypopituitarism; Growth Hormone Deficiency; Pituitary Dwarfism): Growth Hormone Deficiency involves abnormally short stature with normal body proportions. It can be categorized as either congenital (present at birth) or acquired. Normal puberty may or may not occur, depending on the degree to which the pituitary can produce adequate hormone levels other than growth hormone. Synthetic growth hormone can be used for children with growth hormone deficiency. Growth rates are improved in most children treated with growth hormones, although the effectiveness may decrease with prolonged treatment.

Edwards' syndrome (also known as trisomy 18): Trisomy 18 is a syndrome associated with the presence of an extra number 18 chromosome. It is associated with many abnormalities, some of which reduce survival to a few months of life, and few affected babies survive beyond the first year. More than ten children have been known to survive to teenage years, usually with serious handicaps. Complications depend on the specific abnormalities that affect the baby.

Eugenics: The idea of improving humanity by encouraging the strongest and most intelligent to reproduce with the hope of producing better offspring, and/or discouraging the weak and less intelligent from reproducing, thereby minimising the number of 'inferior' offspring. Eugenic principles were behind the Nazi extermination of 'defectives' and eventually the Jews. In the modern era proponents of eugenics have adopted new technological means including birth control, genetic engineering, selective abortion and reproductive technologies.

Foetal tissue transplant: Tissues taken from the bodies of foetuses after miscarriage or abortion and used in experimental therapeutic treatments for conditions like Parkinson's disease. Sometimes the method of abortion is modified to obtain tissues that are more suitable for transplant.

Fragile X (also known as Martin-Bell syndrome, or Marker X syndrome): Fragile X syndrome is a genetic condition involving changes in the X chromosome; it is characterised by mental retardation. Boys and girls can both be affected, but because boys have only one X chromosome, a single fragile X is more likely to affect them more severely. Complications vary depending on the type and severity of symptoms. There is no specific treatment for Fragile X syndrome.

Gene therapy: The treatment of genetic disorders by the manipulation of genes. Harmless viruses are used to introduce a healthy version of a gene into the body to replace a defective version. Somatic gene therapy involves introducing genetic changes that are not passed on to the offspring, whereas germ line gene therapy involves changes to genes that are passed to offspring.

Genes: The units of coded information that give rise to traits. At the molecular level a gene is a segment of DNA on a chromosome arranged as a code made from the sequences of the bases Cytosine, Guanine, Thymine and Adenine. The role of a gene is to manufacture one or more proteins, which are then involved with the generation of a trait.

Genetic engineering: Methods which involve the technological manipulation of genes either to modify a given gene or to transfer a gene from one species to another, or both.

Genetic: Relating to genes and traits.

Germ line therapy: Gene therapy in which genetic changes are made to egg and sperm so that the changes are inherited.

Haemophilia: A hereditary bleeding disorder, affecting mostly males, in which it takes a long time for the blood to clot and abnormal bleeding occurs. The severity of symptoms vary and the severe forms become apparent early on. Bleeding is the hallmark of the disease. Additional bleeding manifestations make their appearance when the baby becomes mobile. Mild cases may go unnoticed until later in life when they occur in response to surgery or trauma. Internal bleeding may happen anywhere, and bleeding into joints is common. With treatment, the outcome is good; most people with haemophilia are able to lead relatively normal lives. A small percentage of people with haemophilia will develop inhibitors of the clotting factor VIII, and may die from loss of blood.

Hereditary: Characteristics transmitted from one generation to the next. In the context of traits, 'hereditary' refers to the transmission of genetic information.

Human Genome Project: Collaborative scientific venture to determine the complete human genetic code. The project was eventually undertaken by two groups in parallel using different methods. The code consists of 3 billion units of information that amounts to approximately 30,000 genes.

Huntington's disease (also known as Huntington chorea): An inherited condition involving abnormal body movements, dementia, and psychiatric problems. It is a progressive disorder caused by wasting (degeneration) of nerve cells in the brain. There is progressive loss of mental function, including personality changes, and loss of cognitive functions such as judgment, and speech. Abnormal facial and body movements develop, including quick jerking movements. (The term chorea means 'dance' and refers to the movements that develop.) Psychiatric illness, depression and suicide are common. There is no known cure or way to stop progression of the disorder. Treatment is aimed at slowing progression and maximising ability to function for as long as possible.

In vitro fertilisation (IVF): Fertilisation outside of the body, typically in a laboratory setting. Hence, in vitro, meaning in glass. Sperm and eggs are collected, and following fertilisation, the embryo develops in a culture medium until, at age 3–5 days, it is transferred to the woman's uterus. If the embryo successfully implants, development continues till birth. The term 'in vitro fertilisation' is often used more broadly to refer to a range of techniques in reproductive technologies.

Induction of labour: A medical intervention designed to artificially initiate contraction of the uterus, leading to dilatation of the cervix and birth of the baby.

Informed consent: A legal condition whereby a person can be said to have given consent based upon a full appreciation and understanding of the facts and implications of any actions (as far as humanly possible), with the individual being in possession of all of her faculties (not mentally retarded or mentally ill), and her judgment not being impaired at the time of consenting (by sleepiness, intoxication by alcohol or drugs, other health problems, etc.).

Karyotype: The chromosomal complement of an individual, including the number of chromosomes and any abnormalities. The term is also used to refer to a photograph of an individual's chromosomes.

MPS-1 (Hurler Syndrome): An inherited disease that belongs to a group of diseases called mucopolysaccharidoses. Storage of abnormal quantities of this material (mucopolysaccharide) in different body tissues is responsible for the symptoms and appearance of the disease. Newborn babies with this defect appear normal at birth but, by the end of the first year, signs of problems begin to show. They slowly develop coarse, thick, facial features, prominent dark eyebrows, cloudy corneas, progressive stiffness, and obvious mental retardation. The disease damages many organs including the heart and heart valves. In the early onset form of the disease, death occurs in the early teens, often from the associated heart disease. Enzyme replacement therapy is now possible for patients with one particular defect. Bone marrow transplantation can improve some of the symptoms of the disease, and to prevent mental retardation, needs to be performed at a very young age. Other treatments depend on the affected organ system.

Mutation: A random change in the genetic code that will be passed on to the next generation. Mutations can result from radiation and chemical damage or occur spontaneously. Most mutations are damaging.

Nanotechnology: Technological methods operating on a very small scale, usually around a millionth of a millimetre. The methods aim to employ tiny machines that could work in environments previously inaccessible.

Neonatologist: A doctor who specialises in the care of sick newborn babies. Physicians must first become paediatricians through three years of specialty training. They then spend another three years sub-specialising in the care of sick newborns.

Neural tube defect: Normally the closure of the neural tube occurs around the 30th day after fertilisation. However, if something interferes and the tube fails to close properly, a neural tube defect will occur. Among the most common tube defects are anencephaly, encephalocele, and spina bifida.

Nuchal Translucency: This is a collection of fluid under the skin at the back of a baby's neck at 10–14 weeks that can be measured using ultrasound. All babies have some fluid, but in many babies with Down syndrome, the nuchal translucency is increased. A nuchal translucency scan is a method of assessing whether the baby is likely to have Down syndrome and can only estimate a risk of the baby having Down Syndrome. It does not provide a diagnosis.

Oxytocin drip: A hormone produced by the hypothalamus and stored in the pituitary gland. It is used to help start or strengthen labour and to reduce bleeding after delivery.

Perinatologist: An obstetrical sub-specialist concerned with the care of the mother and foetus at higher-than-normal risk for complications. Since the perinatal period, depending on the definition, starts at the 20th to 28th week of gestation and ends 1 to 4 weeks after birth, a perinatologist logically could be an obstetrician or paediatrician but, in practice, a perinatologist is an obstetrician.

Placenta accreta: A complication where the placenta attaches deep into the uterine muscle, instead of just on the surface of the uterus. It almost always necessitates a hysterectomy.

Placenta previa: A condition in which the placenta is lying unusually low in the uterus, next to or covering the cervix. Placenta previa is not usually a problem early in pregnancy. But if it persists into later pregnancy, it can cause bleeding, which may require early delivery and can lead to other complications. Placenta previa at the time of delivery, necessitates a c-section.

Preimplantation genetic diagnosis: A diagnostic technique used in the context of reproductive technologies. It involves the removal of one or more cells from a 2–3 day old embryo which are tested for specific genetic characteristics. A decision is then made about the suitability or otherwise of the embryo for implantation. This technique has been used for sex selection, elimination of genetically defective embryos and for the selection of embryos with desired characteristics.

Prenatal genetic diagnosis: Any diagnostic procedure which tests for genetic conditions in the foetus before birth. Prenatal diagnosis involves testing foetal cells, amniotic fluid, or amniotic membranes to detect foetal abnormalities.

Shunt: A device used in the treatment of hydrocephalus, incorporating pipes and valves which are surgically inserted into the head to drain away excess cerebrospinal fluid.

Somatic cell therapy: A form of gene therapy. Gene therapy is the insertion of genes into an individual's cells and tissues to treat a disease, and hereditary diseases in particular. Gene therapy usually aims to supplement a defective mutant gene with a functional one. Although the technology is still in its infancy, it has been used with some success. Somatic gene therapy can be broadly split into two categories: ex vivo (where cells are modified outside the body and then transplanted back in again) and in vivo (where genes are changed in cells still in the body).

Somatic: To do with the body. For example, somatic cells are all body cells other than the germ cells, which are the egg and sperm.

Spina Bifida (also known as Myelomeningocele): A congenital disorder (birth defect) where the backbone and spinal canal do not close before birth. This can result in the spinal cord and its covering membranes protruding from the baby's back. Symptoms are related to where the defect is on the spinal column, and can include partial or complete paralysis of the legs, partial or complete lack of sensation, and may include loss of bladder or bowel control. The exposed spinal cord is susceptible to infection (meningitis). Early surgical repair of the defect is usually recommended, and foetal surgery is now being developed, although surgical repair may be performed later to allow the infant to tolerate the procedure better. Antibiotics may be used to treat or prevent meningitis, urinary tract infections, or other infections. Orthopaedic intervention or physical therapy may be needed to treat musculoskeletal symptoms. Other neurologic damage is treated according to the type and extent of the loss of function. The goal of these interventions is to minimise future disability and maximise functioning. Sometimes surgical shunting to correct hydrocephalus causes the myelomeningocele to spontaneously reduce, and normal growth of the child may cover the defect.

Sterilisation (also known as Tubal Ligation): A surgical procedure commonly known as 'tying the tubes'. A woman's fallopian tubes transport mature eggs from the ovaries to the uterus approximately once a month. Tubal ligation permanently sterilises a woman by preventing transport of the egg (ovum) to the uterus, and by blocking the passage of sperm up the tube to the ovulating ovary where fertilisation normally occurs. Tubal ligation is considered a permanent form of birth control. The operation can sometimes be reversed if a woman later wants to try to become pregnant. However, this requires a major surgical procedure. Following tubal ligation reversal, about 50 percent to 80 percent of women eventually become pregnant.

Surrogacy: An arrangement in which one woman gestates a child for another. The commissioning couple arrange with a surrogate to have a sperm sample from the male partner or from a sperm donor used to inseminate the surrogate. The surrogate mother then gives the child to the couple at birth. Alternatively, the commissioning couple have an embryo of their own or donated, created through in vitro fertilisation, implanted in the surrogate. When born, the child is given to the commissioning couple. Surrogacy arrangements create legal and familial complexities.

Tay-Sachs disease: A familial disorder (it affects more than one member of a family) that results in early death. It is found predominantly in Ashkenazi Jewish families. It is caused by a deficiency of hexosaminidase, an enzyme important in the metabolism of gangliosides which is a type of chemical substance found in nerve tissue. These gangliosides then accumulate in the brain, causing neurological deterioration. Symptoms generally begin to appear when the child is 3–6 months old. The disease tends to progress rapidly, and the child usually dies by the age of 4 or 5 years. There is no treatment for Tay-Sachs disease itself, only ways to make the patient more comfortable.

Trisomy 18: See Edwards' syndrome.

Trisomy 21: See Down syndrome.

Turner syndrome: A genetic condition that occurs only in females. Female cells normally have two X chromosomes. In Turner syndrome, the girl's cells are missing an X chromosome, or part of an X chromosome. There are a variety of signs and symptoms that can result, but the most common are short height, lack of developing ovaries, and infertility. Growth hormone may be considered to help a child with Turner syndrome grow taller. Estrogen therapy is often started in the early teenage years to stimulate the development of breasts, pubic hair, and other sexual characteristics. Those with Turner syndrome can have a normal lifespan when carefully monitored by their doctor.

Ultrasound: A medical diagnostic technique that utilises very high frequency sound waves to 'visualise' structures within the body. The sound waves bounce off internal structures and back to a sensor, which sends the information to a computer to generate an image. Ultrasound is used extensively in obstetrics to view the embryo or foetus throughout development. Recent advances have produced images of very high quality.

Bibliography

ABC (2000, August 23). Genetic supermarkets in the pipeline for family shopping. *7.30 Report*. Sydney: Australian Broadcasting Corporation.

ABC (2001, October 23) Nuchal Screening. *Health Dimensions*. Sydney: Australian Broadcasting Corporation. Available from http://www.abc.net.au/dimensions/health/transcripts/s397857.htm

Abraham, C. (2002, October 26). Gene pioneer urges dreams of human perfection. *Globe and Mail*, Toronto, p. A1.

Abramsky, L., Hall, S., Levitan, J., & Marteau, T.M. (2001, February 24). What parents are told after prenatal diagnosis of a sex chromosome abnormality: Interview and questionnaire study. *British Medical Journal*, 322, pp. 463–466.

Adelaide Advertiser (1992, August 6). New Down's Syndrome test. p.16

Alfirevic, Z., Sundberg, K. & Brigham, S. (2003). Amniocentesis and chorionic villus sampling for prenatal diagnosis. *The Cochrane Database of Systematic Reviews*: 1. Available at http://www.cochrane.org/cochrane/revabstr/AB003252.htm

Allan, G. E. (2001, October 5). Is a new eugenics afoot? *Science*.

Allen, F. (2000, July 7). Shortness is not a death sentence. [Letter to the Editor]. *The Age*, Melbourne, p. 9.

Anastos, K. & Marte, C. (1989). Women – the missing persons in the AIDS epidemic. *Health/PAC Bulletin*, 19(4), pp. 6–13.

Anderson, G. (1999). Nondirectiveness in prenatal genetics: Patients read between the lines. *Nursing Ethics*, 6(2).

Annas, G. J. (1993). *Standard of care: The law of American bioethics*. New York: Oxford University Press.

Arent, L. (1999, August 26). Serving up eggs on the Web. *Wired*.

Armitage, C. (2003, September 6–7). Stretching their legs. *The Weekend Australian Magazine*, pp. 30–33.

Asch, A. (1989). Can aborting 'imperfect' children be immoral? In J.D. Arras & N.K. Rhoden (Eds.), *Ethical issues in modern medicine* (3rd ed.) Mountain View, CA: Mayfield Publishing Co., pp. 317–321.

Bibliography

Australasian Bioethics Information (2003, September 26). British women 'pressured' into aborting disabled babies. *Australasian Bioethics Information 94*. Retrieved 19 June 2005, from http://www.australasianbioethics.org/Newsletters/094-2003-09-26.html

Ball, K. (2003, September 16). 3-month-old girl fights for her life and proves doctors wrong. *The Californian*, San Francisco.

Bartl, A. (2005, April 8). The million-dollar question: Why Eastwood's baby got it wrong. *The Age*, Melbourne, p. 21.

Beech, B. & Anderson, G. (1999). We went through psychological hell: A case report of prenatal diagnosis. *Nursing Ethics*, *6*(3), pp. 250–256.

Begley, S. (1993, December 7). When DNA isn't destiny. *Bulletin with Newsweek*, *115* (5899), pp. 64–65.

Begos, K. & Ingram, D. (2005, April 24). Bill would offer cash reparations to victims of eugenic sterilization. *Journalnow.com*.

Benson, S. (2001a, March 12). Australia: Dark side when life imitates life. *Nationwide News Proprietary Ltd*.

Benson, S. (2001b, March 12). Australia: Human clone trials – Secret DNA cell testing revealed. *Daily Telegraph*, Sydney, p. 9.

Berkowitz, J.M. & Snyder, J.W. (1998). Racism and sexism in medically assisted conception. *Bioethics*, *12*(1), pp. 25–44.

Biesecker, B. (2001, February 24). Prenatal diagnoses of sex chromosome conditions. *British Medical Journal*, *322*, pp. 441–442.

Black, E. (2003). *War against the weak: Eugenics and America's campaign to create a master race*. New York: Four Walls Eight Windows.

Blumberg, L. (1994a, January/February). Eugenics vs Reproductive Choice. *Disability Rag & ReSource*.

Blumberg, L. (1994b). The politics of prenatal testing and selective abortion. *Sexuality and Disability*, *12*(2), pp. 135–153.

Boetzkes, E., Rober, D. & Swanson, C. (2002). Secrecy, integrity, agency: nurses and genetic terminations. *The Journal of Clinical Ethics*, *13*(2), pp. 124–130.

Bouza, T. (1989, May 8). A mother's day wish: Make abortion available to all women. *Minneapolis Star Tribune*.

Boyd, P.A., Chamberlain, P. & Hicks, N.R. (1998, November 14). 6-year experience of prenatal diagnosis in an unselected population in Oxford, UK. *The Lancet*, *352*, pp. 1577–1581.

Boyd, P.A., Tondi, F., Hicks, N.R. & Chamberlain, P.F. (2003, December 8). Autopsy after termination of pregnancy for fetal anomaly: retrospective cohort study. *British Medical Journal*, available at: http://bmj.bmjjournals.com/cgi/content/abstract/328/7432/137

Boylan, E. (1991). *Women and disability*. London: Zed Books.

Brady, S., Briton, J. & Grover, S. (2001). The sterilisation of girls and young women with a disability: Issues and progress. Australian Human Rights & Equal Opportunity Commission. Available at http://www.humanrights.gov.au/disability_rights/sterilisation/index.html

Brennan, F. (2002). The strange logic of 'wrongful life'. *Disparity*, pp. 4–8.

Brookes, A. (1994). Women's experience of routine prenatal ultrasound. *Healthsharing Women*, 5(3&4), pp. 1–5.

Brookes, A. (1998). 'We've got a problem!' Women and prenatal diagnosis: Difficult decisions. Doctoral dissertation, Deakin University, Australia.

Brookes, A. (2001). Women's voices: Prenatal diagnosis and care for the disabled. *Health Care Analysis*, 9, pp. 133–150.

Brooks, L. (1998, December 6). All for the breast. *The Sunday Age*, Melbourne.

Browner, C. & Press, N. (1996). The production of authoritative knowledge in American prenatal care. *Medical Anthropology Quarterly*, 10(2), pp. 141–156.

Buchanan, A., Brock, D.W., Daniels, N. & Wikler, D. (2000). *From chance to choice: Genetics and justice*. Cambridge and New York: Cambridge University Press.

Buck, P. S. (1992). *The child who never grew*. Brentwood, MD: Woodbine Press, 2nd ed.

Burkham, C. (2005, January 15). Nip and tuck nation. *The Age, Good Weekend*, Melbourne, pp. 24–26.

Campbell, F. (2000). Eugenics in a Different Key? New Technologies and the 'Conundrum' of 'Disability'. In M. Crotty, J. Germov, & G. Rodwell (Eds.), *'A race for a place': Eugenics, Darwinism and social thought and practice in Australia. Proceedings of the History & Sociology of Eugenics Conference*. Newcastle: University of Newcastle, pp. 307–318.

Carlson, T. (1996, December 2). Eugenics, American Style: The Abortion of Down Syndrome Babies. *The Weekly Standard*, pp. 20–25.

Carter-Long, L. (2005, February 21). Million Dollar baby – the unasked million dollar question. [Letter to the Editor]. *The Age*, Melbourne, p. 12.

Clarke, A. (1990). Genetics, ethic and audit. *The Lancet*, *335*, pp. 1145–1147.

Clarkeburn, H. (2000). Parental duties and untreatable genetic conditions. *Journal of Medical Ethics*, *26*, pp. 400–403.

Colon, A. (2004, December 3). When killing an infant is not wrong. *The New York Sun*, p. 2.

Conor, S. (2001, April 16). Let us rid society of genetic defects, says DNA pioneer. *Independent*. Retrieved from http://news.independent.co.uk/uk/science/story.jsp?story=66838

Cook, M. (2003, September 29). Human experiments threaten dignity. *Herald Sun*, Melbourne, p. 18.

Cook, M. (2004, Summer). Was this superman really a saint? *Perspective*, p. 28.

Cooper, A. (1995, January 31). Remember what the social engineers wrought. *International Tribune*.

Crotty, M., Germov, J. & Rodwell, G. (Eds). (2000). *'A Race for a place': Eugenics, Darwinism and social thought and practice in Australia. Proceedings of the History & Sociology of Eugenics Conference*. Newcastle: University of Newcastle.

CWNews.com (1998, September 30). Hospital, company sued over abortion decision. *CWNews.com*

Davies, V., Gledhill, J., McFadyen, A., Whitlow, B. & Economides, D. (2005). Psychological outcome in women undergoing termination of pregnancy for ultrasound-detected fetal anomaly in the first and second trimesters: a pilot study. *Ultrasound Obstet Gynecol* 25, pp. 389–392.

de Bruyn, M. (1998). Linking prevention and care in reducing perinatal transmission: What about women? In AZT trials to reduce HIV transmission: A debate about science, ethics and resources – Roundtable. *Reproductive Health Matters*, *6*(11), pp. 129–144.

Dockser M.A. (2002, July 25). Ensuring your baby will be healthy: Embryo screening testing gains in popularity and controversy; Choosing a child's gender. *The Wall Street Journal*, p. D1.

Dunne, A. & Noble, T. (2005, June 5). Should science reshape the human race? *The Sunday Age*, *Agenda*, Melbourne, p. 13.

Dunne, C. & Warren, C. (1998). Lethal autonomy: The malfunction of the informed consent mechanism within the context of prenatal diagnosis of genetic variants. *Issues in Law & Medicine, 14*(2), pp. 165–202.

Duster, T. (1990). *Backdoor to eugenics*. New York: Routledge.

Dymke, K. (2000, July 6). I wouldn't give him up for the world. [Letter to the Editor]. *The Age*, Melbourne, p. 16.

Eide, B. L. (1997). 'The least a parent can do': Prenatal genetic testing and the welcome of our children. *Ethics and Medicine, 13*(3), p. 59.

Elder, S.H. & Laurence, K.M. (1991). The impact of supportive intervention after second trimester termination of pregnancy for fetal abnormality. *Prenatal Diagnosis 11*, pp. 47–54.

Ellingsen, P. (2004, September 26). The seven-year-old looked after in a home for the elderly. *The Sunday Age*, Melbourne.

Ennis, M., Clark, A. & Grudzinskas, J. (1991, September 7). Change in obstetric practice in response to fear of litigation in the British Isles. *The Lancet, 338*, pp. 616–618.

Evans, K. (2003, September 28). Tuesday's child. *The Sunday Age*, Melbourne, p. 4.

Faunce, T. (1998). Perigravid genetic screening: The spectre of eugenics and medical conscientious non-compliance. *Journal of Law and Medicine, 6*(2), pp. 147–167.

Field, B. (1996). Foucault's power/knowledge model applied to genetic screening. Paper presented to 10th World Congress of the International Association for the Scientific Study of Intellectual Disabilities, Helsinki.

Finger, A. (1984). Claiming all of our bodies: reproductive rights and disability. In R. Arditti; R.D. Klein & S. Minden (Eds.). *Test tube women: What future for motherhood?* London: Pandora.

Finger, A. (1990). *Past due: A story of disability, pregnancy and birth*. Seattle: Seal Press.

Finlay, S., Fitzgerald, R. & Legge, M. (2004, June). Cytogeneticists' stories around the ethics and social consequences of their work: A New Zealand case study. *New Zealand Bioethics Journal*.

Finnegan, J. (1991). Relinquishing a child for special needs adoption. Prenatal diagnosis and pregnancy options. *The Genetic Resource, 6*(1).

Fisher, A. (1996). The brave new world of genetic screening: Ethical issues. In J. Flader (Ed.), *Death or disability? Proceedings of a seminar at the University of Tasmania*. Hobart: University of Tasmania, pp. 16–34.

Fitzgerald, J. (2005).Geneticizing disability: The Human Genome Project and the commodification of self.
http://www.metafuture.org/articlesbycolleagues/JenniferFitzgerald/Geneticising%20Disability.htm

Friedlander, H. (1995). *The origins of Nazi genocide: From euthanasia to the Final Solution*. Chapel Hill: The University of North Carolina Press.

Fuhrmann, W. (1989). Impact, logistics and prospects of traditional prenatal diagnosis. *Clinical Genetics*, *36*(5), pp. 378–385.

Fukuyama, F. (2002). *Our posthuman future: Consequences of the biotechnology revolution*. New York: Farrar, Strauss & Giroux.

Furlong, R. & Black, R. (1984). Pregnancy termination for genetic indications: The impact on families. *Social Work in Health Care*, *10*(1), pp. 17–34.

Galton, D. (2001a). *In our own image: Eugenics and the genetic modification of people*. London: Little, Brown and Company.

Galton, D. (2001b). Three Warnings from History. In D. Galton (Ed.). *In our own image: Eugenics and the genetic modification of people*. London: Little, Brown and Company, pp. 69–104.

Gates, E.A. (1994). Prenatal genetic testing: Does it benefit pregnant women? In K.H. Rothenberg & E.J. Thompson (Eds.). *Women and prenatal testing: Facing the challenges of genetic technology*. Columbus: Ohio State University Press.

Germov, J. (2000). 'My Genes Made Me Do It': A Sociology of the 'New Genetics'. In M. Crotty, J. Germov & G. Rodwell (Eds.). *'A Race for a place': Eugenics, Darwinism and social thought and practice in Australia. Proceedings of the History & Sociology of Eugenics Conference*. Newcastle: University of Newcastle, pp. 55–60.

Gevers, S. (1999). Third trimester abortion for fetal abnormality. *Bioethics*, *13*(3/4), pp. 306–313.

Gillam, L. (1999). Prenatal diagnosis and discrimination against the disabled. *Journal of Medical Ethics*, *25*(2), pp. 163–171.

Glover, J. (1990). *Causing death and saving lives*. London: Penguin.

Goggin, G. & Newell, C. (2005). *Disability in Australia: Exposing a social apartheid*. Sydney: UNSW Press.

Gorna, R. (1996). *Vamps, virgins and victims: How can women fight AIDS*. London: Cassell.

Grant, M. (1936). *The passing of the great race*. New York: Charles Scribner's Sons.

Green, J.M. (1993, November 6). Ethics and late termination of pregnancy. *The Lancet, 342*(8880), p. 1179.

Green, J.M. (1994). Serum screening for Down's syndrome: The experiences of obstetricians in England and Wales. *British Medical Journal, 309*, pp. 769–772.

Green, J.M. (1995). Obstetricians' views on prenatal diagnosis and termination of pregnancy: 1980 compared with 1993. *British Journal of Obstetrics and Gynaecology, 102*, pp. 228–232.

Green, J.M., Hewison, J., Bekker, H.L., Bryant, L.D. & Cuckle, H.S. (2004). Psychosocial aspects of genetic screening of pregnant women and newborns: A systematic review. *Health Technology Assessment, 8*, pp. 1–24.

Green, J. M. & Statham, H. (1996). Psychosocial aspects of prenatal screening and diagnosis. In T.M. Marteau & M.P.M. Richards (Eds.). *The troubled helix: Social and psychological implications of the new human genetics*. Cambridge and New York: Cambridge University Press, pp. 140–163.

Greer, G. (1984). *Sex and destiny: The politics of human fertility*. London: Picador.

Griffiths, J. (1999, September 22). Science friction. *The Guardian*. Available at http://www.guardian.co.uk/guardiansociety/story/0,,269788,00.html

Hall, J., Viney, R. & Haas, M. (1998). Taking a count: The evaluation of genetic testing. *Australian and New Zealand Journal of Public Health, 22*(7), pp. 754–758.

Harris, R.A., Washington, A.E., Nease R.F. Jr. & Kupperman, M. (2004). Cost utility of prenatal diagnosis and the risk-based threshold. *The Lancet, 363*, pp. 276–282.

Hawthorne, S. (2002). *Wild politics: Feminism, globalisation and bio/diversity*. North Melbourne: Spinifex Press.

Henderson, M. (2003, July 4). Scientists create mixed-sex embryos. *The Australian*, p. 8.

Hentoff, N. (2005, March 29). Terri Schiavo: Judicial Murder. *Village Voice*.

Hershey, L. (1994, July/August). Choosing disability. *Ms. Magazine*, pp. 26–32.

Hodgson, M. (2005, May 14). A barren choice. *The Age, Good Weekend*, Melbourne, pp. 40–42.

Howe, K. & Frohmader, C. (2001). Going Inclusive: Access to health for women with disabilities. In *Politics, action & renewal: Fourth Australian Women's Health Conference*. Adelaide, South Australia, pp. 199–209.

Hubbard, R. (1986). Eugenics and prenatal testing. *International Journal of Health Services, 16*(2), pp. 227–241.

Hubbard, R. (1987). Eugenics: new tools, old ideas. In E.H. Baruch, A.F. D'Adamo & J. Seager (Eds.). *Embryos, Ethics and Women's Rights: Exploring the new reproductive technologies*. The Haworth Press, New York (also published as *Women and Health 13*(1/2), 1987).

Hubbard, R. (1997). Abortion and Disability: who should and who should not inhabit the world? In L.J. Davis, (Ed.). *The Disability Studies Reader*. New York: Routledge, pp. 187–200.

Hudson, K. (2003, May 3). A warning that must not be ignored. *New Scientist*, p. 5.

Hughes, J. (n.d.). *Democratic Transhumanism*. Retrieved June 15, 2005 from www.changesurfer.com/Acad/DemocraticTranshumanism.htm.

Hunfeld J.A., Wladimiroff J.W. & Passchier J. (1994). Pregnancy termination, perceived control, and perinatal grief. *Psychol Rep., 74*(1), pp. 217–218.

Hunfeld J.A., Wladimiroff J.W. & Passchier J. (1995). The grief of late pregnancy loss. *Patient Education Counselling, 31*(1), pp. 57–64.

Hyler, D. (1985). To choose a child. In S. E. Browne, D. Connors, & N. Stern (Eds.), *With the power of each breath: A disabled woman's anthology*. San Francisco: Cleis Press, pp. 280–284.

Jansen, R.P.S. (1990). Unfinished feticide. *Journal of Medical Ethics, 16*, pp. 61–65.

Johnson, M. (1990, August/September). Aborting defective foetuses – What will it do? *LINK Disability Journal*, p. 14.

Kallianes, V. & Rubenfeld, P. (1997). Disabled women and reproductive rights. *Disability and Society, 12*(2), pp. 203–221.

Kaplan, D. (1998). Disability rights perspectives on reproductive technologies and public policy. In N. Taub & S. Cohen (Eds.). *Reproductive laws for the 1990s: A briefing handbook*. New Brunswick, NJ: Rutgers University Press, pp. 241–47.

Kapuscinski, R. & Popper, K. (1995, January 1). Untitled article in *New York Times Magazine* (Sect 6), pp. 24–25.

Kass, L.R. (1985). *Toward a more natural science: Biology and human affairs*. New York: The Free Press.

Kass, L.R. (1999). The moral meaning of genetic technology. *Commentary*, *108*(2), pp. 32–38.

Kass, L.R. (2002). *Life, liberty and the defense of dignity: The challenge for bioethics*. San Francisco: Encounter Books.

Kent, A. (1974). *The death doctors*. New English Library.

Kerr, A. & Shakespeare, T. (2002). *Genetic politics: From eugenics to genome*. New Clarion Press.

Kersting, A., Reutemann, M., Ohrmann, P., Baez, E., Klockenbusch, W., Lanczik, M. & Arolt, V. (2004, June). Grief after termination of pregnancy due to fetal malformation. *Journal of Pyschosomatic Obstetrics and Gynecology*, *25*(2), pp. 163–169.

Kersting, A., Dorsch, M., Kreulich, C., Reutemann, M., Ohrmann, P., Baez, E. & Arolt, V. (2005, March). Trauma and grief 2–7 years after termination of pregnancy because of fetal anomalies – a pilot study. *Journal of Psychosomatic Obstetrics and Gynecology*, *26*(1), pp. 9–15.

Kevles, D.J. (1985). *In the name of eugenics: Genetics and the uses of human heredity*. New York: Alfred A. Knopf.

Kolker, A. and Burke, B.M. (1993). Grieving the wanted child: ramifications of abortion after prenatal diagnosis of abnormality. *Health Care Women International*, *14*(6), pp. 513–26.

Kolker, A. & Burke, B.M. (1994). *Prenatal testing: A sociological perspective*. Westport, CT: Bergin and Garvey.

Korenromp, M.J., Christiaens, G.C., van den Bout, J., Mulder, E.J., Hunfeld, J.A., Bilardo, C.M., Offermans, J.P. & Visser, G.H. (2005). Long-term psychological consequences of pregnancy termination for fetal abnormality: a cross-sectional study. *Prenatal Diagnosis*, *25*, pp. 253–260.

Koshland, D. (1989). Sequences and consequences of the human genome. *Science*, *246*, p. 189.

Kuebelbeck, A. (2003). *Waiting with Gabriel: A story of cherishing a baby's brief life*. Chicago: Loyola Press.

Kuhse, H. & Singer, P. (1985). *Should the baby live?: The problem of handicapped infants*. Melbourne: Oxford University Press.

Laing, L. (2004, October 23). The baby who would not let go. *Herald Sun*, Melbourne, p. 91.

Lambert, C. (1996a, May 26). Baby scans raise fears. *Sunday Herald Sun*, p. 7.

Lambert, C. (1996b, November 17). Healthy twins nearly aborted after error. *The Sunday Telegraph*, Sydney, p. 37.

Lane, H. (1992). *The mask of benevolence: Disabling the deaf community*. New York: Alfred A. Knopf.

Laughlin, H.H. (1914, January 8–12). Calculations on the working out of a proposed program of sterilization. In *Proceedings of the First National Conference on Race Betterment*, Battle Creek, Michigan, published by the Race Betterment Foundation, pp. 478–494.

Laussel-Riera, A., Devisme, L., Manouvrier-Hanu, S., Puech, F., Robert, Y. & Gosselin, B. (2000). Value of fetopathological examination in medical abortions: Comparisons of prenatal diagnosis and autopsy results of 300 fetuses. *Annales de Pathologie*, *20*, pp. 549–557.

Lawless, S., Kippax, S. & Crawford, J. (1996). Dirty, diseased and undeserving: The positioning of HIV-positive women. *Social Science and Medicine*, *43*, pp. 1371–1377.

Leake, J. & Milich, E. (2001, April 1). Down's test kills more babies than it detects. *Sunday Times*, London.

Lee, M.L. (2004, February). The inadequacies of absolute prohibition of reproductive cloning. *Journal of Law and Medicine*, *11*(3), pp. 351–372.

Leithner, K., Maar, A., Fischer-Kern, M., Hilger, E., Loffler-Stastka, H. & Ponocny-Seliger, E. (2004). Affective state of women following a prenatal diagnosis: predictors of a negative psychological outcome. *Ultrasound Obstetrics and Gynecology*, *23*, pp. 240–246.

Lewontin, R.C. (1997, March 6). Science and 'the demon-haunted world': An exchange. *New York Review of Books*, pp. 51–52.

Liamputtong, P., Halliday, J.L., Warren, R., Watson, L.F. & Bell, R. J. (2003). Why do women decline prenatal screening and diagnosis? Australian women's perspective. *Women and Health*, *37*, 2.

Lifton, R.J. (1986). *The Nazi doctors*. New York: Basic Books.

Lindee, S. & Nelkin, D. (1995). *The DNA mystique: The gene as a cultural icon*. New York: WH Freeman.

Lippman, A. (1991). Prenatal genetic testing and screening: Constructing needs and reinforcing inequities. *American Journal of Law and Medicine, 17*(1&2), pp. 15–50.

Lippman, A. (1994). The genetic construction of testing. In K.H. Rothenberg & E.J. Thompson (Eds.). *Women and prenatal testing: Facing the challenges of genetic technology*. Columbus: Ohio State University Press.

Lloyd, J. & Laurence, K.M. (1985). Sequelae and support after termination of pregnancy for fetal malformation. *British Medical Journal, 290*, pp. 907–909.

Lupton, D. (1999). Risk and the ontology of pregnant embodiment. In D. Lupton (Ed.). *Risk and sociocultural theory: New directions and perspectives*. Cambridge: Cambridge University Press, pp. 59–85.

Madsen, M. (1993, February). Prenatal testing and selective abortion: The development of a feminist disability rights perspective. *STATEing Women's Health*. South Australia: Women's Health Statewide.

Maguire, G. & McGee, E. (1999). Implantable brainchips? Time for debate. *Hastings Center Report, 29*(1), pp. 7–13. Available at http://www.bu.edu/wcp/Papers/Bioe/BioeMcGe.htm

Markens, S., Browner, C. & Press, N. (1999). 'Because of the risks': How us pregnant women account for refusing prenatal screening. *Social Science and Medicine, 49*, pp. 359–369.

Marteau, T.M & Drake, H. (1995). Attributions for disability: The influence of genetic screening. *Social Science and Medicine, 40*(8), pp. 1127–1132.

Meikle, J. (2001, April 2). Down's children denied heart ops by biased doctors. *The Guardian*. BBC News Online. Available at: http://news.bbc.co.uk/1/low/health/1255881.stm

Narasimban, S. (1993, February). The unwanted sex. *New Internationalist*, p. 240. http://www.newint.org/issue240/unwanted.htm

National Centre in HIV Epidemiology and Clinical Research (NCHECR) (2005, January). Australian HIV surveillance report. Sydney: University of New South Wales.

Newell, C. (2002, Winter). Don't deliver us from disability. *Disparity, 1*(1).

Newell, C. (1999). We went through psychological hell: A case report of prenatal diagnosis. *Nursing Ethics*, *6*(3), pp. 250–256.

Noble, T. (2005, June 5). Let us create diseased stem cells – Researcher. *The Sunday Age*, Melbourne, pp. 1–2.

Nolan, C. (1987). *Under the eye of the clock: The life story of Christopher Nolan*. New York: St Martin's Press.

Nolan, K. (1995). First Fruits: Genetic Screening. In J. Howell & W. F. Sale (Eds.). *Life choices: A Hastings Center introduction to bioethics*. Washington DC: Georgetown University Press, pp. 499–505.

Nugent, C. (2004). Grace Anne Nugent's story. Available at http://www.graceannenugent.netforms.com/

Padawer, R. (2005). Sex selection of babies forces new debate. Retrieved June 15, 2005, from http://www.northjersey.com/

Park, J.K. & Strookappe, B. (1996). Deciding about having children in families with haemophilia. *New Zealand Journal of Disability Studies*, *3*, pp. 51–67.

Pence, G. (1998). *Who's afraid of human cloning?* New York: Rowman & Littlefield.

Peter, W.G. (1971, November 15). Ethical perspectives in the use of genetic knowledge. *BioScience*, pp. 1133–1137.

Post, T. (1994, November 29). Quality not quantity. *The Bulletin with Newsweek*, p. 74.

Press, N. & Browner, C.H. (1993). 'Collective fictions:' Similarities in reasons for accepting Msafp screening among women of diverse ethnic and social class backgrounds. *Fetal Diagnosis and Therapy*, *8*(S1), pp. 97–106.

Press, N. and Browner, C.H. (1997). Why women say yes to prenatal diagnosis. *Social Science and Medicine*, *45*(7), pp. 979–989.

Purdy, J. (1999). *For common things: Irony, trust, and commitment in America today*. New York: Alfred A. Knopf.

Purdy, L.M. (1978). Genetic diseases: Can having children be immoral? In John J. Buckley (Ed.). *Genetics now: Ethical issues in genetic research*. Washington DC: University Press of America, pp. 25–39.

Radford, J. (1994). Intellectual disability and the heritage of modernity. In M. Rioux & M. Bach (Eds.). *Disability is not measles: New research paradigms in disability*. North York, Ontario: Roeher Institute, pp. 9–27.

Rakowski, E. (2002). Who should pay for bad genes? *California Law Review, 90*(5), pp. 1345–1414.

Rapp, R. (1988). The power of positive diagnosis: Medical and maternal voices in amniocentesis. In K.L. Michaelson (Ed.). *Childbirth in America: Anthropological perspectives*. South Hadley, Mass: Bergin & Garvey.

Reece, N. (2003), available at
http://www.babiesonline.com/babies/m/micahar/

Reinders, H.S. (2000). *The Future of the disabled in liberal society: An ethical analysis*. Notre Dame, IN: University of Notre Dame Press.

Reuters (2003, July 2). Creation of human 'she-males' sparks outrage. Retrieved from
http://www.ochsner.org/HealthNews/reuters/NewsStory07022003 17.htm

Rhinehart, K.E. (2002a). The debate over wrongful birth and wrongful life. *Law & Psychology Review, 26*, p. 141.

Rhinehart, K.E. (2002b). Legal causes of action for wrongful life are recognized in only three states (California, Washington, and New Jersey). *Law & Psychology Review, 26*, p. 152.

Rifkin, J. (1998). *The biotech century*. New York: Putnam.

Ring-Cassidy, E. & Gentles, I. (2002). *Women's health after abortion: The medical and psychological evidence*. Toronto: The deVeber Institute for Bioethics and Social Research. http://www.deveber.org

Robotham, J. & Smith, D. (2004, August 31). Love me or let me go. *Sydney Morning Herald*. Available at
http://www.smh.com.au/articles/2004/08/30/1093852182205.html

Rosen, C. (2004). *Preaching eugenics: Religious leaders and the American eugenics movement*. Oxford and New York: Oxford University Press.

Rothblatt, M. (1997). *Unzipped genes: Taking charge of baby-making in the new millennium*. Philadelphia: Temple University Press.

Rothman, B.K. (1986). *The tentative pregnancy: Prenatal diagnosis and the future of motherhood*. New York: Viking.

Rothman, B.K. (1989). *Recreating motherhood: Ideology and technology in a patriarchal society*. New York: W. W. Norton.

Rothman, B.K. (1998). On order. In M.C. Nussbaum & C.R. Sunstein (Eds.). *Clones and clones: Facts and fantasies about human cloning*. New York: W.W. Norton, pp. 280–288.

Rowland, R. (1992). *Living laboratories: Women and reproductive technology*. London: Lime Tree/ North Melbourne: Spinifex Press.

Roy, A. (2004, November 7). City of Sydney Peace Prize Lecture. Retrieved June 16, 2005, from http://www.abc.net.au/rn/bigidea/stories/s1232956.htm

Salvesen, K.A., Oyen, L., Schmidt, N., Malt, U.F. & Eik-Nes, S.H. (1997). Comparison of long-term psychological responses of women after pregnancy termination due to fetal anomalies and after perinatal loss. *Ultrasound Obstet Gynecol, 9*(2), pp. 80–85.

Sandelowski, M. & Barroso, J. (2005, May/June). The travesty of choosing after positive prenatal diagnosis. *Journal of Obstetric, Gynecologic, and Neonatal Nursing, 34*, pp. 307–318.

Santalahti, P., Hemminki, E., Latikka, A. & Ryynänen, M. (1998). Women's decision-making in prenatal screening. *Social Science and Medicine, 46*(8), pp. 1067–1076.

Savulescu, J. (1999). Should doctors intentionally do less than their best? *Journal of Medical Ethics, 25*, pp. 121–126.

Savulescu, J. (2005, June 7). It's our duty to make better babies. *Herald Sun*, Melbourne, p. 19.

Schiltz, E. (2004). Living in the shadow of Mönchberg. In E. Bachiochi (Ed.). *The cost of choice: Women evaluate the impact of abortion*. San Francisco: Encounter Books.

Scioscia, A.L. (1999). Prenatal genetic diagnosis. In R.K. Creasy & R. Resnik (Eds.). *Maternal-fetal medicine*. Philadelphia: W.B. Saunders, pp. 40–62.

Shafi, M.I., Constantine G. & Rowlands D. (1988, October 1). Routine one-stage ultrasound screening in pregnancy. *The Lancet, 2*(8614), p. 804.

Shakespeare, T. (1999). Manifesto for genetic justice. *Social Alternatives, 18*(1), pp. 29–32.

Shaw, M.W. (1980). The potential plaintiff: Preconception and prenatal torts. In A. Milunsky & G. J. Annas (Eds.). *Genetics and the Law II*. New York: Plenum, pp. 225–232.

Shaw, M.W. (1984). Conditional prospective rights of the fetus. *Journal of Legal Medicine, 5*, pp. 63–116.

Shildrick, M. (1997). *Leaky bodies and boundaries*. London and New York: Routledge.

Simpson, K. (1992, Summer). Disabled women and health care: The meaning of accessible. *The Women's Foundation Newsletter*, pp. 7–8.

Singer, P. (1979). *Practical ethics*. New York: Cambridge University Press.

Singer, P. (1995, September 16). Killing babies isn't always wrong. *The Spectator*, pp. 20–22.

Smith, J.D. & Nelson, K.R. (1989). *The sterilization of Carrie Buck*. Far Hills, NJ: New Horizon Press.

Smith, W.J. (2003). Continent Death: Euthanasia in Europe. *National Review Online*, http://www.nationalreview.com/comment/smith200312230101.asp

Smith, W.J. (2004). *Consumer's Guide to a brave new world*. San Francisco: Encounter Books.

Sober, E. (2000). Appendix One: The meaning of genetic causation. In A. Buchanan; D.W. Brock; N. Daniels & D. Wikler (Eds.). *From chance to choice: Genetics and justice*. Cambridge and New York: Cambridge University Press, pp. 347–368.

Spallone, P. (1992). *Generation games: Genetic engineering and the future for our lives*. London: The Women's Press.

Stanley, F. et al. (1998, March 12). Doctors fear social backlash. *The West Australian*, p. 5.

Statham, H. & Green, J. (1993). Serum screening for Down's syndrome: Some women's experiences. *British Medical Journal*, *307*, pp. 174–176.

Statham, H. & Green, J. (1996). Psychological aspects of prenatal screening and diagnosis. In T.M. Marteau & M.P.M. Richards (Eds.). *The troubled helix: Social and psychological implications of the new human genetics*. Cambridge and New York: Cambridge University Press.

Stock, G. (2002). *Redesigning humans: Choosing our children's genes*. London: Profile Books.

Strahan, L. (2003, July 11). When 'tis folly to be wise. *The Age*, Melbourne, p.12

Sydney Morning Herald (2001, May 29). Daughter's dash from Pakistan in vain as parliament protestor dies from burns, p. 3.

Tankard Reist, M. (2000). *Giving sorrow words: Women's stories of grief after abortion*. Sydney: Duffy and Snellgrove.

Tankard Reist, M. (2004a). No amount of hand wringing will bring back dead babies after abortion. Retrieved June 17, 2005, from http://www.onlineopinion.com.au/view.asp?article=2560

Tankard Reist, M. (2004b, November 9). So what if the aborted baby cried? Retrieved June 17, 2005, from http://www.onlineopinion.com.au/print.asp?article=2724

Tankard Reist, M. (2004c, November 3). Take a look at late-term abortions. *The Australian*, p. 15.

Taussig, M. (1992). *The Nervous System*. New York: Routledge.

Taylor, Z. (2003, November 10). The price of a baby girl: $14,000 for the chance to choose your child's sex. *Daily Telegraph*, Sydney, p. 6.

Teutsch, D. (2003, March 9). Michelle or Michael? How you can pick sex of baby. *Sun Herald*, Sydney, p. 30.

Thom, D. & Jennings, M. (1996). Human pedigree and the 'best stock': From eugenics to genetics? In T.M. Marteau & M.P.M. Richards (Eds.). *The troubled helix: Social and psychological implications of the new human genetics*. Cambridge and New York: Cambridge University Press, pp. 211–234.

Titmuss, R.M. (1970). *The gift relationship: From human blood to social policy*. London: Allen and Unwin.

Tormey, S. (2004, Winter). Making perfect babies. *Griffith Review*. Retrieved 17 June 2005, from http://www.ozprospect.org/pubs/tormey1.html

Toy, M. A. (2000, July 4). Doctors endorse dwarf abortion. *The Age*, Melbourne. Available at http://www.shortsupport.org/News/0008.html

Toy, M. & Milburn, C. (2000, July 8). Whose life is it anyway? *The Age*, Melbourne, p. 3.

Trombley, S. (1988). *The right to reproduce: A history of coercive sterilization*. London: Weidenfeld and Nicolson.

Truman, R (2001, April 28). A perfect memory of joy, suffering and love. [Letter to the Editor]. *The Age*, Melbourne, p. 6.

Tuch, B.E., Scott, H., Armati, P.J., Tabiin, M.T. & Wang, L.P. (2003). Use of human fetal tissue for biomedical research in Australia, 1994–2002. *Medical Journal of Australia*, *179*(10), pp. 547–550.

Tucker Carlson, E. (1996, December 2). Eugenics American style: The abortion of Down syndrome babies. *The Weekly Standard*, pp. 20–23.

van den Berg, M., Timmermans, D.R.M., Kleinveld, J.H., Garcia, E., van Vugt, J.M. & van der Wal, G. (2005). Accepting or declining the offer of prenatal screening for congenital defects: Test uptake and women's reasons. *Prenatal Diagnosis, 25*(1), pp. 84–90.

Wates, M. & Jade, R. (Eds.). (1999). *Bigger than the sky: Disabled women on parenting.* London: The Women's Press.

Waxman, B.F. (1993). The politics of eugenics. *Disability Rag, 14*(3), pp. 6–7.

Webber, J. (2002). Better off dead? *First Things, 123*, pp. 10–12.

Wendell, S. (1992). Toward a feminist theory of disability. In H.B. Holmes & L.M. Purdy (Eds.). *Feminist perspectives in medical ethics.* Bloomington and Indianapolis: Indiana University Press, pp. 63–81.

Wertz, D.C. & Fletcher, J.C. (1993). A critique of some feminist challenges to prenatal diagnosis. *Journal of Women's Health, 2*(2), pp. 173–188.

Westbrook, M. & Chinnery, D. (1995). The effect of physical disability on women's childbearing and early childrearing experiences. *Australian Disability Review, 3*(4), pp. 3–17.

Wexler, A. (2000). Chorea/graphing chorea: The dancing body of Huntington's disease. In P. Brodwin (Ed.). *Biotechnology and culture: Bodies, anxieties and ethics.* Bloomington and Indianapolis: Indiana University Press.

Wexler, N. (1980). 'Will the circle be unbroken?': Sterilizing the genetically impaired. In A. Milunsky & G.J. Annas (Eds.). *Genetics and the Law II.* New York: Plenum.

White-Van Mourik, M.C.A., Connor, J.M. & Ferguson-Smith, M.A. (1992). The psychosocial sequelae of a second-trimester termination of pregnancy for fetal abnormality. *Prenatal diagnosis, 12*, pp. 189–204.

Whiteside, R.K. & Perry, D.L. (2001). Stereotype, segregate and eliminate: 'Disability', selective abortion and the context of 'choice'. National Council on Intellectual Disability. *interaction, 15*(2).

Wilson, E.O. (1978). *On human nature.* Cambridge: Harvard University Press.

Wolbring, G. (2003, October 12–16). NBIC, NGO's society and three types of disabled people. Paper presented at Heinrich Böll symposium, Within and beyond the limit of human nature, Berlin, Germany.

Wolbring, G. (2004). Disabled people, science and technology and health research. In S. Matlin (Ed.). *Global Forum Update on Research for Health 2005*. London: Pro-Book, pp. 138–141.

Women with Disabilities Australia (WWDA) in Association with the Disability Studies and Research Institute (DSARI) and Lee Ann Basser (2004). Submission to the Commonwealth and state/territory governments regarding non-therapeutic sterilisation of minors with a decision-making disability. Retrieved June 19, 2005, from http://www.wwda.org.au/sterilisesub1.htm

World Transhumanist Association. About the WTA. Retrieved June 19, 2005, from http://transhumanism.org

Wyndham, D. (1997). Striving for national fitness: Eugenics in Australia 1910s to 1930s. Doctoral dissertation, University of Sydney, Australia.

Zamichow, N. (1995, January 10). Newsletter articles stir furore in high-IQ group. *Los Angeles Times*, p. B1.

Zeanah, C.H., Dailey, J.V., Rosenblatt, M.J., Saller, D.N. Jr. (1993). Do women grieve after terminating pregnancies because of fetal anomalies? a controlled investigation. *Obstetrics and Gynecology*, *82*, pp. 270–275.

Zitner A. (2002, July 23). A girl or boy, you pick. *Los Angeles Times*, p. A1.

Index

Vaccination Against Pregnancy: Miracle or Menace
Judith Richter

Judith Richter examines the research into a new class of birth control methods in which the body is challenged by immuno-contraceptives or anti-fertility 'vaccines'. A model book that challenges unorthodox and dangerous research on women's bodies and on their lives. A book that has wrought changes to research and stopped further development of medicines that create harm. Recommended for courses in medical ethics and health.

'Richter's serious and compelling critique of immunological contraceptives . . . is a major contribution to the international women's health movement.'
　　　　　　　　　　　　　　　　　　　　　　　　　—Betsy Hartmann

Women As Wombs: Reproductive Technology and the Battle Over Women's Freedom
Janice G. Raymond

A scathing analysis of high-tech biomedical reproductive techniques. *Women as Wombs* provides groundbreaking insights into the debate over reproductive technology and its ethical, legal, and political implications. She asserts that far from being liberatory issues of 'choice', these techniques – including in vitro fertilization, surrogacy, and sex selection – are a threat to women's basic human rights.

'A strongly written, carefully reasoned critique of the reproductive liberalism that . . . lies behind current concepts of reproductive choice.'
　　　　　　　　　　　　—K. Kaufmann, *San Francisco Chronicle Review*

Wild Politics: Feminism, Globalisation and Bio/Diversity
Susan Hawthorne

Looking for a new way forward? Or a different explanation of what is currently happening? Susan Hawthorne challenges the universal endorsement of global western culture with her concept of biodiversity, arguing that biodiversity is a useful metaphor for understanding social, political, and economic relations in the globalised world of the twenty-first century.

'One of the many gifts of Susan Hawthorne's *Wild Politics* is the unrelenting analysis and illustration of ways neo-colonialism is promoted under the banner of Western liberalism and economic globalization . . . Her goal is to decolonize the Western imagination.'
—Sarah Lucia Hoagland, *Women's Review of Books*

'[*Wild Politics*] is a passionate book offering a kaleidoscope of ideas, arresting ways of seeing things, and possible solutions for many of the man-contrived environmental messes across the violated globe. Its barefaced audacity is its greatest attraction. Hawthorne has blazed a trail for others to follow.
—Alan Patience, 'Best Books of 2002', *Australian Book Review*

Not For Sale:
Feminists Resisting Prostitution and Pornography
Christine Stark and Rebecca Whisnant (Eds.)

This international anthology brings together research, heartbreaking personal stories from survivors of the sex industry, and theory from over thirty women and men – activists, survivors, academics and journalists. *Not For Sale* is groundbreaking in its breadth, analysis and honesty.

'Loving and militant, practical and prophetic, this book collects the least compromised writing on a most crucial problem of our time – even the bottom line issue of all time.'   —Catharine MacKinnon

If you would like to know more about Spinifex Press,
write for a free catalogue or visit our home page.

SPINIFEX PRESS
PO Box 212,
North Melbourne,
Victoria 3051, Australia
http://www.spinifexpress.com.au